More than 90 percent of men and women experience some type of headache at least occasionally. Americans alone spend more then $4 *billion* each year on over-the-counter headache medications. Now, with this one-of-a-kind guide, you can get immediate headache relief using safe and effective natural remedies.

DID YOU KNOW THAT . . .

- Simple breathing exercises release muscle tension and can eliminate head pain?

- Shiatsu can provide significant relief of migraine or sinus headaches, and headaches that accompany colds or flu?

- Acute and recurrent sinusitis can be effectively relieved through acupuncture?

- Hydrotherapy can soothe tension headaches and types of migraines that are accompanied by fever or nausea?

- Reducing salt intake—especially the week before the menstrual cycle begins—can help control headaches that result from increased pressure caused by water retention?

- Magnesium, considered an antistress mineral, can be beneficial in eliminating the head pain of migraine?

DISCOVER THE NATURAL TREATMENT
THAT WILL WORK
FOR YOUR HEADACHE IN

THE *NATURAL HEALTH* GUIDE TO HEADACHE RELIEF

THE 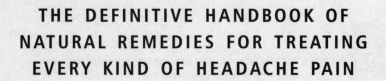 Natural Health GUIDE TO HEADACHE RELIEF

**THE DEFINITIVE HANDBOOK OF
NATURAL REMEDIES FOR TREATING
EVERY KIND OF HEADACHE PAIN**

PAULA MAAS, D.O., M.D.(H.),
DEBORAH MITCHELL,
and the Editors of *Natural Health* Magazine

A LYNN SONBERG BOOK

POCKET BOOKS
New York   London   Toronto   Sydney   Tokyo   Singapore

The ideas, procedures, and suggestions in the book are intended to supplement, not replace, the medical advice of trained professionals. All matters regarding your health require medical supervision. Consult your physician before adopting the medical suggestions in this book as well as about any condition that may require diagnosis or medical attention.

An *Original* Publication of POCKET BOOKS

POCKET BOOKS, a division of Simon & Schuster Inc.
1230 Avenue of the Americas, New York, NY 10020

ISBN: 0-671-51899-2

First Pocket Books trade paperback printing March 1997

10 9 8 7 6 5 4 3 2

POCKET and colophon are registered trademarks of
Simon & Schuster Inc.

Cover design by Tai Lam Wong
Text design by Stanley S. Drate/Folio Graphics Co. Inc.

Illustrations by Dr. Paula Maas

Printed in the U.S.A.

ACKNOWLEDGMENTS

Many people helped in the creation of this book—far too many to name here. My thanks go to Mary Rodriguez, Fravarti O'Hare, Reggie Van Stout, Andy Weil, Bill Nages, Lyn Patrick, Robert Fulford, Marie Schloss, John Dommisse, Jeff Zanderer, and Denise Bey; to my many patients, colleagues, and friends, especially Martin Turner; to my parents; and to the Dalai Lama.

CONTENTS

PART II

NATURAL MEDICINE FOR HEADACHE RELIEF AND PREVENTION

INTRODUCTION

This book can help you open doors to discover natural, safe ways to get headache relief. It can help you identify the causes of your headaches and then introduce you to a comprehensive sampling of natural headache remedies that you can use alone or combine with conventional treatments such as aspirin and other drugs to reduce or eliminate headache pain.

What is *natural?* It is what feels right for you. *Healing* is allowing the body to return to a state of well-being and health. Natural healing occurs in steps, including (1) awareness, which deepens as you discover the factors behind your headache pain; (2) acceptance, in which you reduce any emotional stress you have around your pain, which in turn allows you to see more clearly which healing path is best for you; (3) release, in which you make adjustments to your life style and use the tools that are presented in this book; and (4) commitment, something that is difficult for most Americans, but when you find the cause of your pain you may learn that relief lies in commitment to modifying or eliminating a habit, activity, or attitude.

More and more Americans are turning to natural medicine for headache relief. Their reasons vary, and we discuss these reasons in this book. Many people are like Nancy, who needed a headache therapy that didn't upset her stomach. Nancy's headaches, which occurred about twice a week and lasted a few hours to an entire day, were caused primarily by tension at work. Ibuprofen did not completely relieve her pain, and to make matters worse, the pills made her dizzy and gave her a stomachache. A friend introduced her to a clinical herbalist in her town, who recommended that she drink a tea made of hops and chamomile and also suggested some relaxation methods and exercises to help relieve her stress. Nancy noticed an improvement in her head pain almost immediately. She also began to study yoga and found that the more she practiced, the deeper was her relaxation response and the more easily she could release the stress that caused her pain.

Unlike Nancy, you have the advantage of having this book to help you choose which natural therapies will best relieve your head pain. We suggest you use this book with an open mind and with a sense of adventure and wonder. After you read Part I, start with the techniques that interest you the most. Follow your curiosity. Most of the natural therapies in this book can be used alone or with a partner. Share your experience with someone else, whether it be massage, a movement program, a new eating plan, acupressure, reflexology, yoga, or any of the other techniques we discuss.

This book can help you achieve more than physical relief. It also shows how natural therapies increase self-understanding and how they are self-empowering and healing to the body, mind, and spirit. When you are self-empowered, you are more likely to achieve your goals. Overall healing of the body, mind, and spirit progresses better. Self-understanding may lead you to try therapies you had never considered before.

When you enter the world of natural healing techniques, you can learn to take your time, explore the possibilities, and enjoy the results of your discoveries about yourself. Regardless of which doors you knock on, by opening this book, you have taken the first step toward finding the natural treatment for headache relief that works for you.

PART I

THE NATURE
OF
HEADACHES

1

NATURAL MEDICINE:
A DIFFERENT APPROACH TO HEADACHE PAIN

Headaches are the main complaint behind 80 million doctor appointments made each year in the United States. Americans spend more than $4 billion a year on over-the-counter medications for headaches; this figure does not even include what is spent on prescription drugs.

Many headache sufferers garner relief from nonprescription medications, but many others do not. This book helps you identify the key factors that influence your headache and then presents you with treatment options that go beyond what is found in most headache books. Because much information is already available about what people consider to be standard headache treatment, this book offers you a variety of natural treatments that may complement or replace the conventional medical approaches you have been using. Our goal is to expand your options by showing you the most effective natural therapies for headache pain and explaining how they work. Under no circumstances should you abandon, without the advice of your doctor, any medication you are presently taking. Some medicines, when discontinued abruptly, can cause unpleasant or even serious side effects, including worsening headaches. If you have not consulted a doctor about your headache pain, now is the time to make an appointment. Although you can safely treat most types

3

of headache yourself, it is essential to get a complete physical examination first in order to rule out the possibility that a medical condition is the cause of your headache pain.

NATURAL AND CONVENTIONAL MEDICINE

In this book, we use the term *conventional medicine* when we refer to "standard" or "allopathic" Western medicine, and the terms *natural medicine* or *natural therapy* when we refer to the healing methods described in these pages. (*Holistic* and *alternative* are also sometimes used to describe natural medicine.) Occasionally, we use the term *complementary medicine* to remind you that treatment suggestions in this book are intended to complement and enhance—not necessarily replace—your medical doctor's advice. Indeed, we believe strongly that there is a time and place for both conventional and complementary medicine in today's health-care environment.

The natural therapies explored in this book include homeopathy, herbal medicine, diet and nutrition therapy, chiropractic and osteopathic manipulation, acupuncture, polarity therapy, biofeedback, and meditation, among others. Do these therapies have anything in common? Why are they considered "natural" medicine?

To answer these questions, let's consider some of the characteristics natural therapies share and compare them with conventional approaches. Natural medicine's emphasis is on how to maintain wellness, strengthen various body systems, and prevent disease. Conventional medicine steps in after illness strikes. It focuses on symptoms, cure, and crisis management. Another characteristic of natural medicine is that its practitioners routinely emphasize the role that nutrition, life style, attitude, and emotions play in wellness and healing. Those who practice conventional medicine generally place more weight on the impact of heredity, bacteria, viruses, and parasites on the disease process.

Natural medicine practitioners typically use nonsynthetic products and therapeutic techniques, such as herbs, foods and nutritional supplements, massage, and mind and body relaxation aids, to promote healing and wellness. This approach supports the body's inherent tendency to seek health and well-being. Conventional drugs are synthesized, and the resulting chemicals are typically very powerful and foreign to the body.

A visit to a conventional medicine practitioner usually results in a prescription for drugs that treat symptoms rather than the underlying cause of a particular condition. Natural medicine is based on the idea of holism, which views the individual and his or her ailment as completely interconnected. The term *holism* implies that body, mind, spirit, and emotion are all part of the healing equation, and holistic practitioners consider all these factors and their components—social, environmental, diet, attitude, life style, and stress, for example—as they make a diagnosis and decide on treatment.

The association between mind and body is an integral part of the holistic approach to healing. Mind–body medicine is based on proven clinical evidence that you have the power to influence your health—either positively or negatively—by controlling and redirecting your thoughts and emotions. Techniques such as biofeedback, breathing therapy, self-hypnosis, progressive relaxation, self-talk, meditation, and visualization, discussed in Chapter 7, can help you realize and harness that power. The fact that emotions and attitudes play a significant role in physical well-being has been and continues to be demonstrated by physicians and health-care professionals such as Herbert Benson, M.D.; Joan Borysenko, Ph.D.; Norman Cousins; Deepak Chopra, M.D.; Bernie Siegel, M.D.; and Andrew Weil, M.D. These individuals and countless others who practice and teach natural healing are "reintroducing" us to a power we all possess. (See the Sources and Suggested Readings for books by these individuals.)

In addition to broadening your treatment options by presenting natural therapies, we also want to emphasize that when it comes to conventional physicians and practitioners of natural medicine, it is not a case of "them" versus "us" or "scientific and methodical" versus "humanistic and intuitive." There are good physicians everywhere who provide hands-on comfort and dispense advice that take life-style adjustments into consideration. Many physicians are expanding their education and experience to include homeopathy, acupuncture, bodywork, and various relaxation therapies. There are also both complementary and conventional practitioners who work together to heal a patient: the use of both massage therapy and drug therapy for migraine is an example of this approach.

HOW DO NATURAL REMEDIES WORK?

Each of the many different natural medicine approaches has its own explanation for success. Sometimes our current scientific methods are not able to determine how a particular natural remedy works. However, science is ever-changing, and as quantum physics and different types of energy medicine gain acceptance among scientists and doctors, these new insights may soon reveal explanations for what we now often attribute to the placebo effect.

Although we explain the natural therapies in depth in Part II, here is a broad definition of the four general categories of natural medicine we will discuss.

Nutritional Therapies

Nutritional therapies involve the ingestion of specific plant, mineral, or animal derivatives as well as the addition or elimination of certain foods or supplements in an effort to reduce or eliminate any adverse reactions.

Movement Therapies

Physical exercises and manual therapy by self and others restore and help maintain proper structural alignment and movement patterns so the body can function optimally without compromising the flow of blood, lymph, or bioenergy.

Mind–Body

The goal of mind–body therapies is to achieve inner balance and harmony. The techniques release stress and allow the muscles to relax, and blood pressure and heart rate to fall, digestive juices to flow properly, and emotional tensions to unwind. These changes can occur either through concentrated conscious thought or by allowing the mind to relax.

Bioenergy Therapies

"Every living cell in an organized body is endowed with an instinct of self-preservation which is sustained by an inherent force named *the vital force of life*," is how Henry Lindlahr, author of *Philosophy of Natural Therapeutics*, explained bioenergy. The many disciplines that encompass natural medicine work—some more directly than others—to regain and maintain that vital force, the *qi*, the bioenergy, the flow of energy. It has many names but only one purpose, concluded Lindlahr: "the constant effort of the body's life force is always in the direction of self-cleansing, self-repairing and positive health." Everything we do affects our bioenergy, either indirectly or directly. Acupuncture and polarity therapy unblock the bioenergy flow, for example, without manipulating the body, adding chemicals, or working directly with conscious thought.

HOW DO WE KNOW NATURAL THERAPIES WORK?

Some controlled studies proving the effectiveness of certain natural therapies do exist, but most natural treatments have gained acceptance based on anecdotal evidence. This refers to cases in which people offer their personal experiences with a treatment, rather than data from scientific studies, as evidence and compare their experiences with those of people who have been treated differently. Indeed, many of the natural therapies in this book have been used for thousands of years and have always been a part of pain relief.

Many people rightfully feel that more scientific studies are needed to lend credibility to natural medicine and to garner respect from the conventional medical community. Indeed, there has been a boom in scientific research in many areas of natural medicine. Osteopaths, chiropractors, naturopaths, homeopaths, and other natural medicine practitioners have been publishing results of clinical trials in their journals for many years, although most of the research has been conducted in Europe and other countries.

A step toward bringing that research to the United States has been made by the National Institutes of Health (NIH), which created the Office of Alternative Medicine (OAM) in 1992. According to Joseph J. Jacobs, M.D., director of the OAM when it was initiated, the purpose is to provide physicians and the public with objective "scientific information about the clinical benefits of . . . various procedures." Dozens of grants have been awarded for the study of herbal medicine, chiropractic, acupuncture, biofeedback, and other holistic treatments.

Meanwhile, as research continues, more and more Americans are turning to natural medicine. According to researchers at Harvard Medical School, one of four patients tries natural medicine for at least part of his or her treatment, and one of every 10 patients goes to a holistic practitioner for a principal medical condition, such as headache or high blood pressure.

HOW TO USE THIS BOOK

Although headaches are universal, your headache pain is unique to you. You may experience different kinds of headaches depending on your physical, emotional, and spiritual state at any one time. Your body chemistry and life style are like those of no other person. Therefore, the remedies you choose are for *your* particular needs. How you respond to any given remedy is unique, too. What works for you for one type of headache may not work for another type. Biofeedback and herbal teas may help you but not your spouse or your best friend. That's why this book is structured to help you easily find your headache type and treatment options.

In Part I, you will discover what headaches are and the many factors that influence them. Chapter 2 gives you an overview of headache pain, including how you and your physician diagnose your pain using your detailed history and a physical examination. Chapters 3 through 6 help you to identify your headache type by giving you a brief, comprehensive list of questions. These chapters also discuss the mechanisms of different kinds of headache and refer you to the most effective natural treatments for them.

In Part II, various natural therapies are explained in detail, including how they work, expected results, and how you can apply the treatment yourself, with a friend, or with the help of a health-care practitioner. Chapter 7 includes mind relaxation therapies, including biofeedback, breathing, inner talk, hypnosis, meditation, progressive relaxation, and visualization. Chapter 8 covers the therapeutic benefits of *chi kung/tai chi*, yoga, movement therapies, and posture work. In Chapter 9, we explore bioenergy therapies, including acupressure, acupuncture, Oriental massage, polarity therapy, reflexology, and therapeutic touch. Osteopathic manipulation and other physical therapies, including chiropractic, craniosacral therapy, hydrotherapy, myotherapy, physical therapy, Swedish massage, and transcutaneous electric nerve stimulation, are discussed in Chapter 10. Chapter 11 discusses how dietary and nutritional changes can prevent, reduce, and sometimes eliminate headaches. The worlds of herbal medicine and aromatherapy are explored in Chapter 12, and Chapter 13 looks at homeopathy. Finally, Chapter 14 looks at over-the-counter and prescription drugs, their effectiveness and side effects, and other medical therapies.

At the back of the book is your resource guide for organizations, clinics, and pain centers to contact for more information; sources for herbs, homeopathic remedies, and other products discussed in the book; and natural health practitioners, such as homeopaths, naturopaths, herbalists, osteopaths, licensed massage therapists, and others. If you want more in-depth information about any of the therapies in this book, refer to the Sources and Suggested Readings provided at the end of the book.

We trust this book will help you discover new, natural treatments for your headache pain and, as a bonus, enrich your overall health. There are many safe, natural therapies presented in this book, but only you can choose whether you want to adjust your habits and take a new direction toward health. To help you make the transition to meditation or adoption of a new diet or exercise program as smooth, easy, and fun as possible, we suggest you approach the task with a sense of adventure and enthusiasm. The support of family and friends is important to your success, so share your intentions with them. Take time to explore your options. Choose a technique that feels comfortable to you, fits into your life style, and will be acceptable to others close to you.

The first step is to educate yourself and to work with your physician. We applaud you and encourage your efforts to find headache relief. Once you have succeeded, we hope you will share your success stories with others and help them overcome their pain.

2

HEADACHE:
BASIC QUESTIONS ANSWERED

In simplest terms, a headache is a pain in the head. Headaches may be the most prevalent human symptom. More than 90 percent of people experience some type of headache at least occasionally. Headaches have probably been around since humans first walked the earth. They are mentioned in Babylonian writings dated around 3000 B.C. and in Egyptian papyrus manuscripts. People in some ancient cultures believed demonic supernatural beings were responsible for headache pain, and certainly headaches can hurt like the devil!

Headaches are commonly described as being either acute or chronic. *Acute* headaches involve pain that comes on relatively quickly, can be mild or severe, and last anywhere from several seconds to several days. The term *chronic headache* indicates a pattern of repeated episodes of pain, mild to severe; in rare cases, the pain or ache is continuous. Relief of chronic headaches requires a preventive approach. Most of the techniques in this book can be applied to both acute and chronic headaches. Relaxation techniques, for example, may stop a mild headache from becoming debilitating, and repeated use of these practices may prevent headache recurrence.

Headaches are as unique as the people who have them. They can develop in seconds or creep up slowly. Some headaches flare up for a few seconds or minutes and then disappear; others linger for days. Sometimes the pain can wake you from sleep. The pain may come as pressure or may be throbbing, steady, shooting, tingling, splitting, mild, or strong.

WHAT ARE THE DIFFERENT TYPES OF HEADACHES?

Up to 90 percent of Americans experience the most common headache type—tension or muscle contraction headache. As the name implies, this type of headache occurs when the muscles in and around the head become tense and send pain signals, by several mechanisms, to the temple or other parts of the head. Migraine is the second most common type of headache pain and is believed to affect between 16 million and 18 million Americans. The pain is usually severe and most often confined to one side of the head. Cluster headaches are considered to be the most severe type. They occur primarily in men and, based on the few studies that have been done, in 0.4 to 1 percent of men. These three headache types are discussed in detail in Chapters 3 and 4.

Headaches can also be caused by environmental factors, such as cold weather or loud noise; foods and beverages; hormone changes; prescription and nonprescription drugs; emotions; postural behaviors; dental and jaw problems; vascular (blood vessel) problems; and tumors. Headaches also can accompany fever, high or low blood pressure, lack of oxygen, and infections of the ears, eyes, sinuses, and other structures in the head, or be triggered by physical activities such as exercise, coughing, or sex. Some diseases cause inflammation of various tissues, which can affect the nerves and vessels that supply the nervous system and muscles in and around the head. Head pain that appears after an injury is of particular concern because there is the possibility of bruising and bleeding in and around the brain. If you experience headache after an injury, even weeks after the incident, consult your physician.

Some of the headaches that fit into the categories mentioned above are explored in more detail in Chapters 5 and 6. If you have a diagnosed disease or medical condition that is accompanied by head pain, check with your doctor to be sure the head-ache does not require treatment outside the realm of this book. Although we focus on the management of the common forms of headache, with the guidance of your doctor, many of the thera-pies we present can bring pain relief from some of the more unusual headache types.

THE HEADACHE WHEEL

The headache wheel (Figure 2-1) illustrates some of the many influences and factors that are likely contributing to your head-ache. Which ones do you believe play a part in your head pain? Which factors would you like to learn more about? Are there any influences and factors that you immediately dismiss as irrel-evant? These may be the very ones that hold the key to pain relief for you. How would you draw your headache wheel, and which factors would be supporting your pain? We have included only a few of the many possibilities, yet these suggestions may help you determine which influences and factors are specific to you.

We suggest that you draw your own headache wheel. Begin with the basic circle and add the "spokes" or factors you think contribute to your headache. As you read through the rest of the chapters in this book and learn more about your type of head-ache, add or change factors as you discover them. This approach will enable you to choose the treatments most likely to relieve your headache pain.

You have the power to affect the factors that cause your head-ache, and you probably are already doing so instinctively. Whenever you have head pain and you dim the lights, tell your family you've got a headache, take medication, lie down, put an ice pack on your forehead, or rub your sore muscles, you address various influences and add or adjust certain factors. These and other natural techniques of pain relief are discussed in Part II.

WHO GETS HEADACHES?

Almost all of us get headaches at one time or another. Head-aches affect males and females, young and old, regardless of

The Headache Wheel

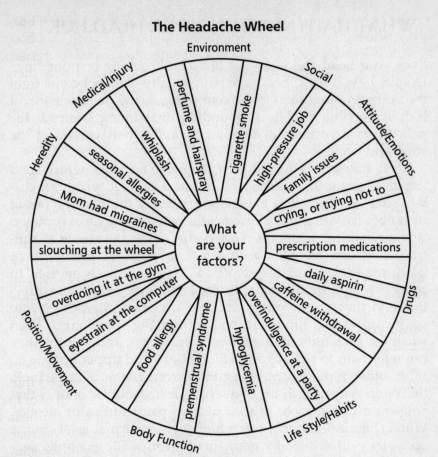

Figure 2-1
The headache wheel provides a visual way to help you consider major influences and discover specific factors that may contribute to your headache pain. It also illustrates that headache pain is a complex, multifactorial condition. The wheel reproduced here is only an example. Your own headache wheel will look different.

socioeconomic, cultural, or educational background. There are differences in prevalence within different headache types, however. Women, for example, are more likely to have migraines or tension headaches than men, while more men than women suffer from cluster headaches. Another type of headache that affects more men than women is cough headache, which is severe pain that occurs upon coughing, bending, sneezing, stooping, or lifting.

WHAT HAPPENS WHEN YOUR HEAD HURTS?

Does your head feel like your brain is throbbing or pounding? Despite how it feels, headache pain usually does not come from the brain. In more than 99 percent of cases, the pain, whether it is dull, piercing, throbbing, pounding, or stabbing, begins in the pain fibers associated with muscles and blood vessels of the scalp and neck.

Pain arises from irritation of the nerve endings, which send impulses along their cell fibers to referred areas, which are distant sites at which you experience pain. Of the many types of pain fiber irritation that cause headache pain, the most common is a mechanical irritation. This occurs when a muscle is contracted, which happens with stress or postural problems, or when muscles are overstretched, as with whiplash injuries. In cases of whiplash, for example, the head is thrown in one direction and then in the other, and the stretched muscles go into spasm to restore alignment and protect the spinal cord. Even when the neck muscles are not noticeably sore and painful, they can refer pain to various parts of the head and upper body.

Another type of irritation comes from chemical substances that occur naturally in the body, such as histamines, or ones that you are exposed to or ingest, such as paint fumes or alcohol. When chemical irritants reach higher than normal levels in the body, they effect pain by many mechanisms. For example, they can change the size of blood vessels and so affect blood pressure and heart rate as well as nerve function and brain activity. To learn which irritants may be causing your headache and how to eliminate them from your life, see Chapter 6.

WHY DO HEADACHES HAPPEN?

Sometimes you can easily identify a single factor as a direct cause of your pain. One young woman began experiencing chronic headache with her new job as a gasoline attendant and got relief only after she quit. For 3 agonizing months, she had breathed fuel and exhaust fumes every day. Other factors may have had some effect on her pain, yet in this case, it made the most sense to address the obvious factor first.

For most people, however, headache is an accumulation of several influences and factors. These influences and factors will become evident to you as you read the following chapters and create your own headache wheel. For example, factors such as stress and food intolerance are very common contributors to headache pain. To find out if they are causing your head pain, you can turn to Chapters 3, 4, and 6. Medical conditions such as arthritis and injuries such as whiplash also are frequently associated with headache. A discussion of medical conditions linked with headache pain is presented in Chapter 5.

WHAT ARE THE DIFFERENT CATEGORIES OF HEADACHE?

This book looks at four basic headache categories: tension headaches; vascular, involving contraction and expansion of the blood vessels in the head, as in migraine and cluster headaches; those caused by environmental, hormonal, or life-style factors; and headaches caused by disease or other medical conditions. Our primary focus is on the first three groups, as they make up the vast majority of headaches that people experience. The last group includes headaches caused by an underlying disease or injury, such as a fever, a blow to the head, a brain tumor, secondary inflammation, infection, or a metabolic, chemical, or vascular problem. The majority of headaches in this category are not serious. To determine whether your headache may be part of a medical condition, or if you are concerned that your headache may be serious, see Chapter 5 and contact your physician.

There is much overlap between headache types, and one type of pain can trigger another type. In Chapters 3 through 6, there are lists of typical characteristics to help you quickly identify your headache. These guidelines are useful only in that they allow you to more readily distinguish the factors unique to your head pain. Choose the description that best describes your pain, read the rest of the chapter to learn which influences and factors are usually associated with that type, and which natural therapies are recommended. You are referred to specific sections in Part II, where an in-depth description of these therapies is presented.

As you read about the different influences and factors that can be involved in headaches, you will see that it is very common to have a "mixed" headache type. If stress is the primary influence on your headache, for example, you may presume you have a "tension headache" and choose stress reduction as your treatment. Let's say your headache is normally accompanied by a stuffy head and is relieved by a decongestant. If you avoid dairy products for a week and the stuffiness goes away, you may consider the headache to be "food related." However, elimination of dairy foods is just one factor you have altered. Influences from other headache types also can affect your headache type. Look openly at all the possible influences so you don't miss important factors, even those you think are unlikely candidates in causing your pain. When you use the headache wheel to explore your headache, you can break away from the limits set by headache type guidelines. The guidelines are a starting point; the wheel allows you to move across the lines of influence and explore *your* pain pattern.

HOW ARE HEADACHES DIAGNOSED?

If you experience an occasional headache and can confidently point to stress or premenstrual syndrome (PMS) or indulgence in a chocolate bar as the cause, you probably do not need to see a physician. Many people diagnose and treat headache successfully on their own. We do recommend, however, that you see a doctor to rule out any serious underlying causes for your pain before you start any self-treatment. Some of the therapies in this book are powerful and can increase your tolerance for pain to the extent that you may be coping with a condition that requires surgery or other conventional treatment. Again, seek professional advice if you have any concerns about your head pain.

HEADACHE DIARY

Pain is a personal and subjective thing; thus, it is difficult to describe and quantify. We recommend using a *headache diary* to help make your task easier. A headache diary is a simple way to comprehensively identify the influences that surround your awareness of pain, target the factors that contribute to it, and compare the intensity and depth of your pain in relation to other possibly influencing factors. This method can help both you and your doctor diagnose and treat your headache. For the diary to be useful, we recommend several things:

- Make it portable: a small notebook or datebook that fits in your purse or pocket is convenient.
- If you don't feel like writing when you have a headache, make a mental note of your thoughts and feelings and jot them down before you forget.
- Be honest. Whether you are doing the diary for your own use only or for a physician, don't hide or deny information about your smoking or drinking habits, fights with your girlfriend, drugs you may be taking, or times you were humiliated at work. All of these factors can have a significant impact on your headache.
- Be creative and specific when you explain your pain. Use words or draw pictures that will remind you of the sensation and intensity.

A sample blank diary page appears on page 18. Use the questions in the accompanying box "Questions for Yourself" (page 19) to help you fill in your diary. You may need to keep notes for several headache episodes to see a pattern and to keep track of variables such as food, exercise, medication use, and so on.

WHAT HAPPENS IN THE DOCTOR'S OFFICE?

After reviewing your diary or asking you similar questions (see Questions the Doctor May Ask, page 20), your doctor will conduct a physical examination. Let your doctor know your questions and concerns even before the examination begins. The more comfortable you feel with the doctor, the more effective your interaction will be. Good communication between the two of you builds good rapport and a trusting, caring relationship. This is an important part of healing.

Following are some common aspects of a physical examination:

- *Temperature measurement:* Headache and fever are a common combination in colds and flu, ear infections, tonsillitis,

Headache Diary

Day and Date	Time Pain Started	Trigger or Situation	Location of Pain	Severity* from 1–10	Duration of Pain	Description of Pain	Other Symptoms	Treatment/ Action Taken	Response to Treatment

*Rate severity of pain from 1 (very mild) to 10 (completely debilitating)

QUESTIONS FOR YOURSELF

- Where is the pain located? One or both sides of your head, behind your eyes, in your temples, in the back of your head?

- Describe the pain: is it sharp, dull, throbbing, stabbing?

- Is the pain constant or does it come and go?

- Do you have pain at regular intervals, such as time of day or with your menstrual cycle?

- What time of the day does the pain first start?

- How long does the pain usually last?

- Does the pain come on suddenly or build slowly?

- Do your headaches seem to be triggered by any of the following: certain foods, beverages, or activities such as exercise or a certain posture at work? (Leave extra space to consider each category separately.)

- How do you usually treat your headache? How do you respond to these treatments?

- Do you smoke, drink alcohol or caffeine products, or use drugs? How much?

- What treatments or remedies have you used for your headache—recently and in the past?

- Are you now going through or have you recently been through a period of great stress?

chest infections, sinusitis, urinary infections, mononucleosis, pneumonia, and gastroenteritis. Many other less common ailments also are associated with fever and headache
pain.

- *Blood pressure measurement:* High blood pressure is a cause
  of headache in some individuals.
- *Heart rate:* An irregular, slow, or rapid heartbeat may be
  a sign of fever or of cardiac, metabolic, or other medical
  problems.
- *Growths, lesions, muscle tenderness, inflammation, or any other
  abnormalities of the neck and head:* These may indicate the
  cause of headache. For example, tender neck muscles or
  temples are common in tension headache; swelling and
  sensitivity of the temporal artery is characteristic of temporal arteritis (see Chapter 5). The doctor also may feel for
  trigger points, which are areas that cause you to feel a sudden jolt of pain when they are touched. Trigger points are
  discussed in more detail in Chapters 9 and 10.

QUESTIONS THE DOCTOR MAY ASK

- When did you first get the headache?

- Do you have any unusual symptoms along with or before the headache,
  such as dizziness, weakness, fuzzy thinking or grogginess, vision problems (such as jagged colors or lights, spots in front of your eyes, blurred
  vision), fatigue, sensitivity to light or sound, numbness, tingling in your
  arms or legs, nausea, vomiting, sleepiness, personality changes, ringing
  in your ears, or trouble thinking or remembering?

- Do you have a family history of headache?

- What is your history of headache? Do you remember having headaches
  as a child?

- Did you ever have a head or neck injury?

- Have you had any dental work done recently?

- Did your friends or family notice any personality changes before or after
  your pain started?

- *Examination of the ears, nose, and throat:* The doctor will check these areas, especially for congestion or the pressure of thick, sometimes odorous mucus running down the back of the throat, which indicates sinus infection. Tapping on the forehead and cheeks may reveal sinus congestion or infection, and a bulging membrane in the ears may indicate ear infection. Some doctors use a small flashlight or x-rays to detect sinus congestion.
- *Examination of vision:* An eye examination can reveal glaucoma, signs of diabetes or hypertension, and inflammation, as well as changes in vision, which is a common cause of headache.
- *Skin examination:* Pimples, boils, and other skin problems over the face and scalp can contribute to head pain.
- *Dental and jaw problems:* Cavities, abscesses, gum disease, clicking jaw, misaligned bite, or tender jaw joints, as in temporomandibular joint (TMJ) syndrome, are frequent causes of headache.
- *A neurological examination:* This includes tests of eye–hand coordination, gait, and reflexes and a series of tests on the 12 cranial nerves. An abnormality of any of these nerves may indicate that part of the brain is not working correctly. Results of a thorough physical examination will alert the physician to any abnormalities or suspicious conditions, in which case he or she may order additional tests. If you do need more tests, it does not necessarily mean something is seriously wrong. Physicians order these tests to rule out certain conditions as well as to confirm any suspicions. The results help them make a more accurate diagnosis.

What Tests Might Be Conducted?

Here are some of the tests and the reasons they may be ordered.

COMPUTED TOMOGRAPHY SCAN

PURPOSE: Computed tomography (CT) is used to detect brain injuries or abnormalities that may be an indication of stroke, tumor, or infection. WHERE: These scans are performed in a radiology laboratory or hospital by a technician, nurse, or doctor. PREPARATION: Do not eat or drink for 12 hours before the test.

Disrobe, remove all jewelry, and put on a hospital gown. RISKS: Emits less radiation than conventional x-rays. Some CT scans are done with a relatively harmless injectable dye that allows the structures to be detected better. This dye contains a type of iodine that can cause a reaction in people who are allergic to shellfish. TIME: The scan takes approximately 30 to 45 minutes. WHAT TO EXPECT: You will lie on a table that slides inside the CT body scanning unit. A computer-controlled scanner revolves around your head and takes multiple x-rays of your head. Beyond having to lie still, there is no discomfort. If you are claustrophobic, keep your eyes closed and breathe slowly. You may take calming herbs or a mild sedative before the procedure.

MAGNETIC RESONANCE IMAGING

PURPOSE: Magnetic resonance imaging (MRI) is done to confirm diagnoses of suspected diseases of the soft tissue of the brain and spinal cord, including tumors and brain swelling. It may be ordered instead of a CT scan, depending on several factors, as MRI is better able to detect certain details than is CT. WHERE: MRI is performed in the hospital by a technician or physician. PREPARATION: There are no food, drink, or activity restrictions. Disrobe, remove all jewelry, and put on a hospital gown. RISKS: MRI cannot be performed in women who have a metal intrauterine device (IUD) or individuals who have a pacemaker or any metal implants, such as artificial hips or pinned fractures. Dental implants and fillings are not a problem. TIME: The MRI takes approximately 45 minutes. WHAT TO EXPECT: You will lie on a table that slides inside the scanner. The scanner uses a magnetic field and radio energy to produce images of your brain. You will not feel these fields or energy waves. If you are claustrophobic, keep your eyes closed and breathe slowly. You may take calming herbs or a mild sedative before the procedure.

ANGIOGRAPHY

PURPOSE: Angiography is used to detect abnormal blood circulation and blood vessel changes that may be caused by tumors, hemorrhage, or dilation of blood vessels. WHERE: Angiograms are performed in the hospital, doctor's office, or radiology laboratory by a technician, nurse, or physician. PREPARATION:

Do not eat or drink for 12 hours before the test. Disrobe, remove all jewelry, and put on a hospital gown. RISKS: This procedure is not recommended for individuals with some types of liver, kidney, or thyroid disease. If it is done on an outpatient basis, arrange to have someone drive you home. Angiography has been used less often since the introduction of CT and MRI, which have less risk, less discomfort, and offer similar information. However, for individuals with suspected blood vessel problems such as an aneurysm (a weakening and ballooning of an artery), an angiogram provides superior images of the blood vessels, which physicians need to determine treatment strategy. TIME: This procedure takes 20 to 45 minutes. WHAT TO EXPECT: You will lie on a table with your head held still. After anesthesia is applied, a dye is injected into an artery. A series of x-rays is taken rapidly. POST-TEST PRECAUTIONS: Rest for 12 to 24 hours. Watch for swelling at the injection site and apply an ice pack if necessary. If the injection was made in an arm or leg, immobilize that limb for 12 hours.

LUMBAR PUNCTURE (SPINAL TAP)

PURPOSE: A lumbar puncture confirms the presence of meningitis, brain abscess, brain hemorrhage, and other life-threatening conditions and measures cerebrospinal fluid pressure. This test is important because it allows physicians to determine if an infection may be causing the head pain. Lumbar puncture is usually indicated in cases in which people report having the most severe headache in their life or having a new headache accompanied by neck stiffness, a suspicious rash, or a change in mental status. Normal cerebrospinal fluid is clear; cloudy fluid suggests possible infection; bloody fluid indicates a hemorrhage. A small amount of blood in the fluid is normal and comes from the surrounding small blood vessels. WHERE: Lumbar puncture is performed in the hospital, radiology laboratory, or doctor's office by a physician. PREPARATION: There are no restrictions; disrobe. RISKS: To help prevent headache after the procedure, you must lie flat on your back without your head raised for 12 hours. Drink plenty of fluids. About 25 percent of people experience a headache after lumbar puncture despite taking these precautions. TIME: The tap takes 30 to 45 minutes. WHAT TO EXPECT: You will lie on a table on your side with your knees drawn up to your chin or you may sit bent forward, which opens up the space between your vertebrae. You will need to remain still throughout the procedure. The injection site will be sterilized and local anesthesia will be injected into the tissues overlying your spine. The physician will then insert a needle into the space that contains spinal fluid. Both the injection and the needle cause some discomfort, which you can control using relaxation techniques (see Chapter 7).

BRAIN SCAN

PURPOSE: Brain scans are done to detect brain tumors or abnormalities in brain structure or function. WHERE: Scans are performed in a nuclear medicine laboratory, hospital, or doctor's office by a physician, technician, or nurse. PREPARATION: There are no restrictions; disrobe, remove jewelry, and put on a hospital gown. RISKS: Brain scans cause no side effects except possible bruising or swelling at the injection site. The procedure involves less radiation than you get with a standard x-ray, and the radionuclides (radioactive chemicals) soon decay into harmless materials. TIME: The procedure takes approximately 45 to 60 minutes. WHAT TO EXPECT: You will lie on a table, and a radioactive chemical called a radionuclide will be injected, usually into the arm. This material travels to the brain, where it emits gamma rays, which are similar to x-rays. A scanner is positioned near your head and detects the rays emitted from the radionuclide in your body. Besides the quick injection, you won't feel a thing. This procedure is simple but its use has declined with the increased use of CT.

Although it is natural to be apprehensive when you undergo tests such as those explained above, the results can offer peace of mind, as they allow both you and your physician to better understand your condition and what may be causing your headache pain. In those rare instances when a medical condition is at the root of your head pain, test results provide your physician with the information she or he needs to help offer you relief.

So far, you have read about some of the physical aspects of headache pain, and we have referred you to appropriate sections in this book for more details. Now we turn to explanations of the different headache types in the next four chapters.

3

TENSION/MUSCLE CONTRACTION HEADACHES

Tension headache is the most common kind of headache there is. Also referred to as muscle contraction or stress headache, it affects three times more women than men and tends to run in families. If you have tension headache, you're not alone: most people experience a tension headache at least occasionally, and more than 80 percent of the people who visit their doctors complaining of headache have this headache type.

Answer the questions about tension headache in the box on page 26. Some of the questions can apply to other headache types, too. It is rare for head pain to be a pure example of one headache type. The questions below and those in the three subsequent chapters are an attempt to identify your *primary* headache type so you can better treat it.

DO YOU THINK YOU HAVE TENSION HEADACHE?

If you answered yes to five or more of the questions in the box entitled "Could It Be Tension Headache," you probably suffer from tension headache. That may not sound definitive enough, yet experts with the Headache Classification Committee of the International Headache Society (IHS) continue to grapple with a "good" definition. For now, it stands as this: "an ache or sensation of tightness, pressure, or constriction, widely varied in intensity, frequency, and duration, sometimes long-lasting and commonly suboccipital [occurring in the lower part of the back of the head]."

Distinguishing tension headache from migraine also may not always be easy or even necessary. You may find that as you go through the influences on the headache wheel (see page 13) and try different techniques, you can relieve your pain regardless of the exact diagnosis. Many people seem to suffer from both headache types, which can make it difficult for physicians to draw a clear line between them. To avoid confusion, the questions posed in this and subsequent chapters are based on the criteria established by the Headache Classification Committee.

COULD IT BE TENSION HEADACHE?

How would you describe your headache pain?

- As if there is a tight band around your head?

- As a dull, aching feeling?

- As if someone or something were squeezing your head?

- As more annoying than severe or incapacitating?

- Located usually in the temples, forehead, or back of the head and neck and relieved by neck or shoulder massage?

Are your headaches accompanied by frequent or early awakenings?

Do your headaches occur during times of tension, depression, conflict, or anxiety and then go away when the stressful situation is over, or occur after a stressful period has passed?

Does the pain usually occur without other symptoms, such as nausea, vomiting, or sinus congestion? Tension headaches frequently occur without accompanying symptoms.

Until a better understanding of the causes and mechanisms of all headache types is reached, this is the system most physicians use to diagnose headache.

There are two types of tension headache: episodic and chronic. Not all experts agree on the definition of these two types. The IHS defines episodic headache, the most common of the two types, as that which occurs less than 15 days per month. If tension headache pain sends you running for the aspirin bottle every day on a regular basis, you may have the chronic type. We discuss chronic tension headache below. In either case, now is the time to explore the influences that contribute to your pain and to try a few techniques to find relief naturally.

IS THERE A "TENSION HEADACHE TYPE"?

If tension headache affects so many people differently, how can we categorize it? Some researchers have formed generalizations about headache types and emotions. These characteristics are not meant to pigeonhole you into a category but to offer possible insight into a cause for your headache pain.

For example, some researchers found that about one-third of the people they questioned with tension headache also have symptoms of depression. Others have found that people who get tension headaches also tend to be energetic and meticulous and have a strong will to succeed. They were said to harbor feelings of doubt and inadequacy. Unresolved anger or guilt, along with anxiety about any number of things—work, school, a relationship, and so on—were also noted. Whether having certain personality traits or emotions predispose people to headaches remains far from clear, but it is safe to say that emotional and physical stress contribute to tension headache. Awareness and release of emotional factors can help relieve headache, especially when the situations that worsen headache are avoided.

WHAT CAUSES TENSION HEADACHES?

Ask 20 people what triggers their tension headache and you *should* get 20 different answers, yet most people will simply say "stress" without being specific. Some of the answers they could give include sitting for long periods of time at a desk; fighting with their children, spouse, or boss; depression; speaking in front of an audience; frustration; trouble falling asleep; financial troubles; worrying about their school grades. All of these situations represent some kind of stress—physical or psychological— yet all are very different, just as every person and his or her headache is unique.

Physical Causes

Several mechanisms may explain the physical cause of tension headache. One occurs when muscles in the head or neck, or both, contract in response to a physical or an emotional trigger. The muscle contraction squeezes the surrounding blood vessels and deprives the tissues of sufficient blood and oxygen; it also irritates the nerves themselves. The tissues then release pain-causing biochemicals, such as histamine, serotonin, and brady-kinin, and pain sensitizers, such as prostaglandins. Then the nerve fibers in the area send the pain signals to the brain, and you experience head pain. A typical muscle tension headache, for example, is one in which the occipital muscles in the back of the neck squeeze the nerves and create head pain.

Trigger Points

Another explanation of tension head pain focuses on the importance of trigger points, tight bands within the muscles of the head, upper back, and neck where nerves and blood vessels are squeezed. When these areas are touched with finger pressure, the nerves may send pain signals from that spot to another in the head and cause headache pain. A trigger point located on the neck muscles just above the collar bone, for example, is one of the most common sources of muscle contraction headache. Another common spot is at the top of the shoulder, in the trape-zius muscle.

Muscle Contraction

Most tension-holding patterns are not apparent to others, but some are. Do your friends ever tell you that you always look worried or that you often frown or look intense? Do you clench your fists or grind your teeth? You may be tensing up muscles in your face, neck, and jaw without realizing it. This constant muscle contraction may be the cause of your tension headaches.

Temporomandibular Joint

Another cause of tension-type headache is misalignment of the jaw or spasm of the muscles of the jaw, called the temporomandibular joint (TMJ) syndrome. This is a very common condition: between 10 million and 14 million people in the United States have TMJ syndrome, and between 60 and 80 percent of them are women. Approximately 50 percent of people with TMJ syndrome have headache as their primary complaint. You may have this condition if you can answer yes to these questions:

- Are your jaws tired when you wake up in the morning?
- Do you grind and clench your teeth especially at night?
- Does it hurt when you move your jaw from side to side?
- Do you have difficulty chewing?
- Do you hear a clicking or popping sound in your jaw when you chew?
- Are your jaw joints or surrounding muscles tender when you touch them with your finger? The surrounding muscles attach to the jaw joint, which is located about one half inch in front of the ear canal.
- Are you unable to open your mouth wide enough to place three fingers between your teeth?
- Do your jaws ever feel like they are locked?
- Are the muscles around your ears, jaw, and temples painfully tight?

Another cause of TMJ syndrome is poor bite due to tooth decay, misalignment, or injury to the jaw or teeth. Uneven wear of the teeth and misalignment may have a genetic origin, but in most cases, they are due to "torquing of the jaws," caused by stress and habit. This is good news because there are exercises and techniques that can relieve the pain. Clicking or locking of the jaw joint may be related to TMJ headache, but it also occurs often in people without this disorder. People who have headache associated with TMJ syndrome may also have ringing in the ears, nausea, dizziness, loss of balance, and sensitivity to light.

Chronic Daily Headache

Head pain that occurs every day or nearly every day and lasts for days, weeks, months, or even years, is considered chronic daily headache. Many factors can trigger this type of headache pain, including TMJ syndrome, eye problems, sinus disorders, and emotional issues, such as stress, depression, and anxiety. Many people who have chronic daily headache also have signs of depression: fatigue, sleep problems, appetite changes, and low sexual desire.

One of the most common causes of chronic daily headache is habitual, long-term use of pain medications. People who experience this type of headache pain typically begin by having one or two headaches a week, which they usually treat with aspirin and acetaminophen. These headaches may be caused by any of the triggers mentioned above. After several months, the drugs are not effective and the headaches begin to come more frequently. Some headache sufferers then often turn to prescription medications, which also frequently become ineffective over time. By this point, headache is a constant part of their life, and each day, they take several times the recommended dose of pain relievers, both prescription and nonprescription, in an effort to get relief. Many people with chronic daily headache take these drugs for months or years.

If you have a similar pattern of headache pain and medication use, you are likely experiencing *rebound headache*, head pain caused by the use of the very drugs you are taking to stop the pain. Treatment consists of gradual withdrawal from these medications, and some people require hospitalization to help them in this process. The use of homeopathic and herbal remedies, as well as practice of some relaxation techniques, can be helpful during the withdrawal process.

Chronic daily headache, as we have said, also may be triggered by many other factors. If your job involves detail work or looking at a computer terminal much of the day, chronic eye strain may be behind your headache pain. Likewise, continuous pressure in the head from sinus conditions or chronic muscle tension caused by a highly stressful life style are also causes of chronic headache pain. Regardless of the cause of the pain, chronic headache is usually relieved once the underlying cause is addressed or treated—for example, withdrawal from medications, stress-reduction therapy, treatment for TMJ syndrome, or relief from eye strain.

HOW TO PREVENT AND TREAT TENSION HEADACHE

To reduce or eliminate the recurrence of tension headache, we recommend you choose a treatment strategy. Creating your own headache wheel (see page 13) is an effective way to discover the factors that are contributing to your tension headache pain. If you think you have tension headache, making your own headache wheel can be an effective way for you to uncover the causes of stress in your life. Do you have a job that requires a lot of detail work, decision making, danger, or other stressful situations? Is there tension between you and your spouse, friends, co-workers or supervisors, or family? Do you have financial or marital problems? Are you worried about job security? These and dozens of other situations can cause tension headache. Once you identify the factors, you can choose natural approaches to prevent and treat your tension headache pain. Review the questions at the beginning of this chapter (see page 26) and then think about how your life style may be contributing to your headache pain. Or you may find that keeping a headache diary (see page 18) works best for you because it allows you to track which situations seem to trigger headache pain. Once you have created your headache wheel or completed a headache diary, you may find the unique combination of situations that cause your headache pain and become aware of the most appropriate treatment options.

In the chapters that follow, you will find therapeutic options for tension headache associated with physical and emotional stress, including help for insomnia, which often accompanies headache.

- *Chapters 7, 8, 9, and 10:* All therapies are appropriate.
- *Chapter 11:* See The Healthiest Eating Plan.
- *Chapter 12:* See Black Cohosh, Catnip, Devil's Claw, Feverfew, Ginseng, Hops, Lavender, Oat, Passionflower, Peppermint, Scullcap, Valerian, White Willow; for insomnia, see Hops, Oat, Passionflower, Valerian.
- *Chapter 13:* See gelsemium, euphrasia, silica.
- *Chapter 14:* See Acetaminophen, Nonsteroidal Anti-

inflammatory Drugs. For chronic headache prevention, see Antidepressants.

Tension headache is a very individual condition: it can be triggered by many different types of stress, and how you react to any given stressful situation may differ from time to time, depending on other factors in your life at the moment. We invite you to explore the therapeutic options presented in this chapter that best match your unique headache situation.

4

MIGRAINE AND CLUSTER HEADACHES

Does your headache pain make you want to creep into a dark room, close the door, and pull the covers over your head so you can block out the world? Does your head hurt so much you feel sick to your stomach and sometimes vomit? Do you experience throbbing, one-sided pain in your head? These are some of the characteristic symptoms of migraine, a type of vascular headache. A *vascular* headache involves the abnormal narrowing (constriction) and expansion (dilation) of the blood vessels within and around the skull. Cluster headaches are another type of vascular headache; we discuss them later in this chapter.

In the next few pages we will help you determine whether you have ever experienced migraine or cluster headaches and then suggest various natural therapies for both types. Answer the questions about migraine in the box on pp. 35–36. The more yes answers you have, the more likely it is that you have the headache type described. Although neither migraines nor cluster headaches are dangerous conditions on their own, it is best to have your self-diagnosis confirmed by a physician to make sure your pain is not associated with a more serious problem.

TYPES OF MIGRAINE

Between 20 and 30 percent of all people with migraine experience classic migraine. This type of head pain is characterized by the *aura stage,* which is marked by symptoms that develop over a 5- to 20-minute period and typically precede the head pain by less than 60 minutes. Have you experienced any of these symptoms of the aura stage?

- Visual disturbances, such as spots in front of the eyes, zigzag lines, blind spots (similar to the blindness caused by a camera flashbulb), tunnel vision, or other visual distortions.
- Pins-and-needles sensation anywhere in the body, such as the arms, legs, face, and tongue; sometimes it affects the entire side of the body

Most people with migraine have it without aura (also called common migraine). The only significant difference between the two types of migraine is the absence of the aura stage in common migraine. Both types of migraine have similar pain and symptom patterns during the preheadache stage (also called the *prodromal stage*) and the headache stage.

If you answered yes to at least three of the questions in the box on pp. 35–36, you may be among the 15 to 20 percent of American men or the 25 to 30 percent of American women who get migraines. The incidence of migraine peaks between 20 and 35 years of age and then gradually declines.

IS THERE A "MIGRAINE TYPE"?

Some physicians believe that people who get migraine share certain personality characteristics. Dr. Uwe Henrik Peters, director of the Neuro-Psychiatrische Universitatsklinik in Mainz, Germany, finds that people who are orderly, precise, and conscientious about their work or schooling are likely candidates for migraine. He also says the "migraine type" has difficulty relaxing. These generalities are not meant to force people into rigid categories. Rather, identifying one or more of these traits in yourself may prompt you to take a different view of yourself and how these traits affect your head pain.

COULD IT BE MIGRAINE?

The questions below refer to both classic and common types of migraines.

During the prodromal stage, which can occur anywhere from a few hours to a few days before the headache phase, do you experience any of the following (not all migraine sufferers experience this stage)?

- Mental symptoms, such as depression, euphoria, irritability, restlessness, hyperactivity, talkativeness, drowsiness.

- Increased sensitivity to sound, odors, light, or touch.

- Neurological symptoms, such as tingling or numbness on one side of the body, staggering walk or incoordination, mental confusion or cloudiness, slurred speech, trouble finding the right word to say, or inability to speak at all. These same symptoms can also indicate a serious condition, such as stroke, and require immediate evaluation the first time you experience them.

- Cold hands or feet caused by constricted blood flow.

- Stiff neck, excessive thirst or urination, fatigue, pale skin, food cravings, diarrhea, or constipation. These symptoms also can occur with other headache types but may be part of the migraine prodromal stage.

Is the headache stage characterized by any of the following symptoms?

- Pain that begins as throbbing on one side of the head.

- Pain in the forehead, eyes, both temples, or top of the head.

- Pain in the jaw or one nostril.

Do you experience any of the following along with your head pain?

- Nausea and/or vomiting.

- Paleness.

- Constipation or diarrhea.

- Oversensitivity to light or sounds.

- Overall muscle achiness.

- Oversensitivity to touch on the face, scalp, and neck.

- Chills and/or fever.

- Muscle spasms in the back and neck.

Before the pain subsides, do you urinate more than usual?

Does the pain last anywhere from several hours to three days?

Once the headache is gone, do your muscles ache or do you feel exhausted or mentally confused?

Is there a history of migraine in your family?

Did you experience recurrent vomiting, stomachaches, or motion sickness as a child? (More on this below.)

Robert is a person who demonstrates some of these traits. His co-workers can always count on him to attend to every last detail of a presentation. He is a terrific "right-hand person" and is a whiz at organizing and implementing plans from behind the scenes. He works tirelessly, both at his job as an architect and at home on the weekends, when he does custom woodworking and often works past midnight to perfect a project. In the office, they jokingly call him "Iron Man" because his blueprints are so sharp and crisp they look like he ironed them. His migraines appear when he is winding down from a project or a busy week at home and at the office. This phenomenon is common among many migraine sufferers. The prevailing theory is that as soon as these individuals begin to relax after a period of stress, worries and anxieties emerge from their subconscious, triggering a migraine. When they are busy, they can avoid emotional pain by distracting themselves with activities. Once the distractions stop, the tension is expressed as a migraine.

There is no consistent "migraine type," and many people with the above characteristics do not suffer from migraine. The role of stress and how individuals handle stress are clearly essential influences in migraine. There is also evidence that the tendency to have migraine is inherited (see The Gene Connection, below), or learned (subconsciously) from one's family.

WHAT CAUSES MIGRAINE?

We wish there were a simple answer to the question of what cause migraines. Most migraines probably begin in the cortex (the outer brain layer) where thoughts are processed. They also have chemical triggers. It is believed that an initiating substance or event, such as coffee, stress, or hormonal changes, triggers an irregular pattern of electrical activity in the cortex. This disturbance causes the prodromal symptoms that sometimes occur before a migraine. Studies show that during this preheadache stage, excessive constriction of the arteries inside the skull (intracranial) reduce the blood flow to the brain.

Some consider the beginning of the headache stage to be when the blood vessels inside the skull squeeze, or constrict, and force an increase in blood flow to the vessels in the face and scalp. This increased blood flow can last for more than 48 hours and may be accompanied by the prodromal symptoms mentioned above. After the initial constriction of the blood vessels inside the head, there is a rebound effect, which means the blood vessels inside the skull expand. Individuals who take medications to constrict the blood vessels before this rebound stage can get migraine relief.

For some people, migraine pain is triggered by environmental toxins such as automobile exhaust or paint fumes; for others, it may be stress; hormone imbalance or fluctuations, such as occur during the menstrual cycle; dietary influences, such as monosodium glutamate (MSG) or caffeine; or sleep disruptions. Any of these factors, alone or in the right combination, may cause migraine.

On a biochemical level, there is an increase in the level of several neurotransmitters (substances that carry messages from one nerve to another) in the preheadache stage. One of these substances, serotonin, causes blood vessels to constrict and also regulates pain and mood. Other substances, such as substance P, are likely involved in the rebound effect and in causing pain, swelling, nausea, and other migraine-related symptoms.

The Gene Connection

Twelve-year-old Mark got his first migraine when he was 10. His mother was not surprised; she has had migraines since she was 21, and her mother gets them, too. New research suggests a strong case for a genetic cause for migraines. Researchers have known for some time that a family history is one risk factor for migraine. Studies in the 1960s, for example, showed that 50 to

60 percent of people with migraine had parents who also had migraine. A search for the responsible gene or genes is now being conducted. Steve Peroutka, M.D., of San Francisco reported in spring 1994 that his study of family members with migraine shows a clear-cut genetic link. He continues to look for the "major, major gene" he believes is responsible for most of the migraine experience.

Be assured, however, that just because one or both of your parents suffer with headache does not mean you will automatically have headaches, too. The genetic connection is only one influence in your headache wheel.

WHAT TRIGGERS A MIGRAINE?

Like the proverbial straw that breaks the camel's back, migraine is often triggered by what appears to be one incident but is actually an accumulation of several factors. Following are some of the many factors that may trigger or exacerbate migraine pain.

Hormonal Changes

The changes in hormone levels that occur before and during menstruation, pregnancy, menopause, and when taking contraceptive pills or other hormone therapy can trigger migraine. (See more details in Chapter 5 under Hormone-Related Headache.) Generally, women who are susceptible to migraine and who take birth control pills or estrogen therapy need to have their estrogen/progesterone doses monitored and altered if these substances increase or cause migraine. Tell your gynecologist or family doctor about any migraine pain.

Hypoglycemia

An abnormally low blood sugar level—hypoglycemia—can occur when you increase your exercise or activity level, decrease your food intake by skipping meals or fasting, get too much sleep, or have an excess of insulin in the blood stream. These situations can trigger migraine pain as well as other types of headaches. Severe hypoglycemia is characterized by sweating, nervousness, early-morning headache, fatigue, foggy thinking, and an emotional slump several hours after meals, especially those including sugary foods. Hypoglycemia occurs frequently among people with diabetes who take more insulin than they need for their calorie-exercise balance. Foods that cause sensitivity or true allergic reactions also may be involved, in which case you may need to identify the culprits and eliminate them from your diet (see Chapter 11).

Hypoglycemia can usually be prevented by eating frequent, healthy meals or snacks. If your headaches occur during the night, have a complex carbohydrate snack (such as whole-grain crackers or a bagel) before going to bed.

Hypertension

Because high blood pressure can cause headache, those who have both hypertension and headache often have more frequent attacks. If you fit into this category, do not take over-the-counter medications that contain a decongestant such as phenylephrine or pseudoephedrine (e.g., Sudafed); also avoid prescription drugs that contain amphetamines, such as diet pills. Headaches can result from any mood-altering substance, from caffeine to alcohol. Cocaine is particularly dangerous for people with hypertension because it can cause headache as well as sudden death from heart attack. The following high-blood-pressure medications may also cause headache: hydralazine, minoxidil, nifedipine, prazosin, and reserpine. In addition, avoid the herbs licorice and ephedra. Some physicians also recommend that women who have hypertension not take estrogen, but it is frequently prescribed when the doctor and the patient believe the benefits outweigh the risks. (Also see Chapter 5 under Hypertension.)

Physical Stress

Many situations fall under the category of physical stress, and any one or more may trigger headache if you are susceptible. These include too much or too little sleep, a sudden change in eating patterns, high humidity, rapid changes in the weather, overexertion or sudden increase in exercise activity, a mild blow to the head, poor ventilation, and exposure to strong odors or excessive noise, light, heat, cold, or motion. (Also see Chapter 6 under Environment-Related Headaches and Life Style/Physical Stress–Related Headaches.)

Allergy

During certain types of allergic reactions to food, beverages, or drugs, the histamine levels in the body increase. Histamines are a group of chemicals that are present in all our cells. They activate stomach acids, are involved in the immune and inflammatory processes, and cause blood vessels to swell, including those in the head. In individuals who are susceptible, the result often is headache, sometimes accompanied by nausea and stomach pain. Other types of food allergies lead to a more chronic but less dramatic reaction: they worsen migraines by triggering digestive problems and by causing antibodies to react with nerves, blood vessels, muscles, and most body tissues. Food allergy is far more common than once thought and is separate and additive to food intolerances (see below).

Food and Drug Intolerance

Results of various studies show that anywhere from 30 to 93 percent of people who have migraines have an intolerance to certain substances present in specific medications, beverages, and foods, such as the amino acid tyramine, which is found in aged cheeses; sodium nitrite, a preservative used in hot dogs and other processed meats; or MSG, a flavor enhancer found in many foods. A discussion of how these substances can cause headache and what you can do to uncover and manage hidden food intolerances is presented in Chapter 11.

Emotional Stress

Tension, stress, and anxiety can trigger not only tension headaches but migraines, too, in people who are prone to migraine, as explained above (under What Causes Migraine?).

MIGRAINE IN CHILDREN

Migraine in children is not uncommon and is sometimes overlooked. By age 15, 5 percent of adolescents have experienced a migraine attack. Boys are more affected than girls up to the age of puberty, and then girls are affected more often, an apparent association with the start of menstruation. Toddlers who vomit frequently may be experiencing migraine pain that they cannot yet express in words. It is not until they are older and can verbalize the pain that parents or physicians make the connection and can diagnose early childhood migraine. Migraine is usually diagnosed in children when headache is on only one side of the head, there are visual disturbances before the pain begins, and there is nausea and vomiting. Seventy percent of children with migraine have a history of this headache type in their family.

Think back to when you were 7 or 8 years old: did you have stomachaches, vomiting, periods of dizziness, or severe motion sickness? Some researchers believe that for many adult migraine sufferers, these nonheadache complaints were actually early symptoms of migraine.

PREVENTION AND TREATMENT OF MIGRAINE

Use the questions presented at the beginning of this chapter (see pp. 35–36) to help you determine which factors are contributing to your migraine pain. Create a headache wheel (see page 13) or keep a headache diary (see page 18). Once you have identified the causes of your pain, you can try several of the natural approaches presented below to help prevent and treat your migraine pain.

Many individuals enjoy migraine pain relief when they combine natural approaches that work together to provide balance to the entire body and to relieve pain. Migraine pain associated with the menstrual cycle, for example, is also often accompanied by breast swelling, weight gain, and food cravings, especially for chocolate. A natural healing approach for this type of migraine may include a prescription from your osteopath for natural progesterone, available in various forms, that normalizes the estrogen-to-progesterone ratio; magnesium for the chocolate cravings and calcium to balance the magnesium; and a decrease in salt intake and supplementation with vitamin B_6 and dandelion leaf, which are mild diuretics, to help with weight loss.

Perhaps you have completed your headache wheel and believe your work environment, diet, and stress are all factors contributing to your migraine pain. What approaches should you take? These factors have already been discussed in this chapter; review them now and then turn to the chapters that address these factors in depth.

In the chapters listed below, you will find natural therapies that serve several purposes. Some prevent pain; that is, they avoid clear triggers such as foods that can initiate migraine; some, like relaxation techniques, reduce the effect of cumulative triggers to a point below your threshold for headache attack. Some treatments reduce the severity of pain and some can cure it; acupressure, posture therapy, and the manipulative therapies, for example, may cure some people and bring partial relief to others.

- *Chapters 7, 8, 9, and 10:* All therapies are appropriate.
- *Chapter 11:* See Elimination Diet Plan, The Healthiest Eating Plan, and Nutritional Supplements as Treatment.
- *Chapter 12:* See Dong Quai, Feverfew, Fringe Tree, Ginseng, Guarana, Peppermint, White Willow, and the Combination Remedies box.
- *Chapter 13:* See belladonna, bryonia, euphrasia, glonoinum, and natrum muriaticum.
- *Chapter 14:* See Acetaminophen, Ergot Alkaloids, Beta-Blockers, Calcium Channel Blockers, Antidepressants, Narcotic Analgesics, and Sumatriptan.

CLUSTER HEADACHES

Cluster headache affects approximately 1 million Americans compared with the 16 million to 18 million Americans who have migraine. You may be among that 1 million if you answer yes to three or more of the questions on page 43, especially if you smoke. Most cluster headache patients are free of pain for months or even years between attacks. About 20 percent of people with cluster headaches, however, experience chronic pain, which means they do not have long pain-free periods between attacks. This is a rare condition and is sometimes treated with surgery.

ARE YOU THE CLUSTER HEADACHE TYPE?

If you are a man, you are eight to ten times more likely than a woman to have cluster headache. A sketch of a typical cluster headache patient was composed by J. R. Graham, M.D., who

COULD IT BE CLUSTER HEADACHE?

Do you experience the following symptoms or have the following characteristics?

- Is the pain isolated to one side of the head and behind your eye?

- Does the eye on the affected side droop and look puffy?

- Is the pain excruciating? Cluster headache pain can make an otherwise stable individual consider suicide.

- Is the pain steady rather than pulsing or throbbing?

- Is the pain accompanied by sweating, blurred vision, and tearing of the eyes?

- Does your nose get stuffy and runny?

- Do you smoke cigarettes?

- Do you drink alcohol regularly?

- Are you male?

- Are you between the ages of 20 and 50?

- Was the first occurrence of this pain after your teenage years?

- Do the headaches occur in clusters of one to three a day over a few days and always occur at the same time?

- Do the headaches recur every few months or even years?

- Do the headaches usually wake you up 2 to 3 hours after you go to bed?

- Does the pain begin suddenly, without warning?

- Do you tend to be tense, anxious, or frustrated?

paints a picture of a tall, rugged, muscular man with a Kirk Douglas dimple in his chin or a square, jutting jaw. Behind the haze from the two packs or more of cigarettes a day he smokes—more than 90 percent of Americans with cluster headache are heavy smokers—you will probably see hazel eyes. He drinks more alcohol than he should and tends to be anxious, aggressive, frustrated, and tense. On a positive note, he is conscientious, self-sufficient, and responsible. Both women and men with cluster headache often have coarse skin that resembles an orange peel. It is unclear why these traits are particular to people with cluster headache, although heavy tobacco use, which directly affects blood vessels and nerves, may play a role we don't yet understand.

WHAT TRIGGERS CLUSTER HEADACHES?

The same triggers that set off migraine are responsible for triggering cluster headache: emotional stress; certain foods or beverages, especially alcohol; and biochemical or hormonal changes in the body. Tobacco use is a consistent influence in cluster headache and should be eliminated.

WHAT HAPPENS DURING A CLUSTER HEADACHE?

Like migraine, cluster headaches are characterized by expansion and constriction of blood vessels and also likely involve changes in serotonin levels. Unlike migraine, however, cluster headaches occur in a cyclical pattern, which some believe implies a disruption or malfunction in the body's biological clock. Our biological clock regulates the sleep–wake cycle, body temperature, enzyme activities, hormone production, and other physiological functions. Both serotonin and histamine, substances that affect the blood vessels, help regulate the biological clock. Changes in the levels of these two substances, together or separately, may have a role in causing cluster headaches. For now, the exact cause of cluster headaches is unknown. Statistics do not indicate that susceptibility to cluster headaches is inherited.

PREVENTION AND TREATMENT OF CLUSTER HEADACHES

The lack of warning and the tendency to begin in the middle of the night make cluster headaches hard to treat. The most important things you can do, however, are reduce stress and eliminate smoking and alcohol from your life style.

Although cluster headaches occur without warning, there are

several preventive and treatment steps you can take. Refer to the designated sections in the following chapters.

- *Chapters 7 and 8:* All therapies are appropriate.
- *Chapter 9:* Acupressure/Shiatsu, Acupuncture, Polarity Therapy.
- *Chapter 10:* Craniosacral Therapy, Myotherapy, Physical Therapy, Transcutaneous Electrical Nerve Stimulation.
- *Chapter 14:* Nonsteroidal Anti-inflammatory Drugs, Ergot Alkaloids, Calcium Channel Blockers, Antidepressants, Narcotic Analgesics, Corticosteroids, Other Drugs, Medical and Surgical Interventions.

Those who experience the usually severe headache pain associated with migraine or cluster headaches often experience some pain relief when they practice natural healing approaches. To enjoy the greatest benefit, we suggest you use a combination of life-style changes and physical and bioenergy therapies that best suit your needs and interests.

5

HEADACHES WITH MEDICAL CAUSES

This chapter is not meant to frighten you. In fact, it may help ease some fears. Are you the type of person who says, "I know I have a brain tumor" every time you get a headache? Or do you have chronic headache pain but won't have it checked because you are afraid the doctor will find something wrong?

First, it is appropriate to fear the unknown. Fear is natural and can be relieved with information and appropriate action. Second, less than 10 percent of all headaches in Americans have an underlying medical problem that is causing the pain. The category "medical causes" includes something as simple as a bump on the head or the common cold. Third, less than 5 percent of all headaches in Americans are related to a *serious* illness, such as a brain tumor. These facts do not mean that headaches with medical causes are any more or less painful than other headaches; they can be just as mild or as severe. It does mean, however, that because there may be an underlying problem that requires treatment, we recommend that you consult a physician for a diagnosis.

Scores of medical conditions can be accompanied by headache, and it is not always easy to distinguish between head pain that is or is not associated with disease. If you have been diagnosed with a medical condition that is associated with headaches, you may find the illness in the sections below, which refer you to specific natural therapies. We divide these medical conditions by type—inflammatory and autoimmune, infections, injury, pressure, neurological, hormone-related, and other for those that don't fit anywhere else—and discuss several of the more common conditions.

If you suspect a medical condition but are afraid you will get a disturbing diagnosis, please make an appointment today. Your decision to seek medical help does not mean you will end up undergoing an endless cycle of expensive tests and procedures. Rarely do visits to a physician for headache result in further testing, and those that do can lead to the discovery of a lesion or other complication early rather than late. In addition, good physicians respect their patients' right to know about and take part in their treatment every step of the way. Once you have given a thorough medical history and had a physical examination, your physician usually can determine whether you have an underlying medical condition, and you can decide on your treatment course together.

As a general note, natural therapies can complement and frequently replace conventional medical approaches in medical conditions accompanied by headache. Holistic treatments can lessen the pain and tension imposed by the influences we've seen on the headache wheel, such as stress, emotions, environment, life style, diet, and others, and promote more effective healing. To help you decide whether your headaches may be associated with a medical condition, answer the questions in the box on page 48.

MEDICAL CONDITIONS THAT CAN BE ASSOCIATED WITH HEADACHES

Below are some of the more common medical conditions that may be accompanied by headaches. There are many more, but they tend to be seen less frequently.

DO YOU HAVE . . . ?

- . . . daily or almost daily headaches? Most of the time, these headaches are chronic tension or mixed tension-migraine headaches, but if yours is getting progressively worse in intensity and/or frequency, please have it checked.

- . . . progressive resistance to medications that once provided you relief? This situation can creep up on you. For example, at one time, 500 mg of ibuprofen relieved your pain; now you take 1,000 mg each time but get little or no relief.

- . . . headaches that wake you up in the middle of the night? This is typical of tension headaches as well as migraines and cluster headaches, but it also can indicate the presence of an infection, intracranial pressure, hypoglycemia, severe hypertension, sleep apnea, or other conditions.

- . . . confusion, memory loss, dizziness, mood swings, double vision, significant weakness, temporary loss of consciousness, seizures, or problems with coordination? Any of these symptoms may indicate a serious condition.

- . . . headaches accompanied by fever? Both headaches and fever are common characteristics of flu, sinusitis, and other nonserious viral infections, but they also are associated with more serious infections, such as meningitis.

- . . . headaches that come on suddenly and/or are unusually intense or excruciating, especially after exertion? This pain is significantly different from the more mild headache commonly brought on by becoming overheated by strenuous exercise.

- . . . headaches that began after age 50 or headaches that are much more severe than any you experienced before 50? This may indicate temporal arteritis or other serious disease associated with middle or later years.

- . . . headache after a fall or blow to the head? Subdural hematoma (a mass or clot of blood) is a possibility after even a minor head injury among people of any age, but especially among the elderly.

INFLAMMATORY AND AUTOIMMUNE DISEASES

Inflammatory conditions such as arthritis, cervical spondylosis, multiple sclerosis, systemic lupus erythematosus (SLE), and temporal arteritis are often accompanied by headache. These are all examples of autoimmune diseases, which involve the body's immune system attacking its own cells as if they were a foreign substance. This in turn causes inflammation and, often, headache.

Temporal Arteritis (Giant Cell Arteritis)

Inflammation of the temporal artery of the scalp is called temporal arteritis ("itis" means "inflammation"). Headache occurs in about 85 percent of individuals with this condition. Temporal arteritis is often accompanied by pain and weakness primarily in the shoulders, hips, and thighs and also in the neck in a syndrome called polymyalgia rheumatica. Temporal arteritis rarely affects people younger than 55 years of age and occurs twice as often among women as among men. Head pain typically occurs daily and on both sides of the head. Pain may be throbbing and sometimes burning. The pain is usually less intense when you sit upright and worse when you lie down or stoop over. Double vision or loss of vision, sensitive scalp, and pain in the jaw when chewing are other presenting signs. *Treatment:* Temporal arteritis is not a condition you should treat on your own, as it has the potential to cause blindness if not treated with medication. See Chapter 10, Physical Therapy (range-of-motion exercises, heat, and hot packs), for pain and weakness; and Chapter 14, Corticosteroids, for temporal arteritis.

Arthritis and Cervical Spondylosis

Arthritis means inflammation of the joint tissues. Cervical spondylosis is a type of arthritis in which bony deposits form on the spine. The neck muscles are usually tender and sometimes cause limitation of neck movement. Up to 80 percent of people with cervical spondylosis experience headache, which usually resembles tension head pain and is located at the back of the head.

Frequently headaches are attributed to problems with the neck joints when an individual's x-rays indicate wearing down or irregularity of the joint surfaces. Conventional treatment occasionally includes surgery, but sometimes natural therapies can bring significant relief. The extent of degeneration seen on x-rays does not necessarily correlate with the severity of symptoms. Degenerative joint disease, for example, frequently appears without symptoms. Also, people with neck or headache pain caused by muscle spasm may inappropriately attribute it to joint pain. A case in point is Martha, an 80-year-old woman who had sharp neck and head pain every time she moved her neck. She was wearing a cervical collar on her first visit to an osteopath. During that visit, she learned to relax her neck muscles and was able to turn and bend her neck in all directions. During her second visit, she learned to stand, sit, and otherwise move without her typical pain. She immediately canceled the surgery she had scheduled for the following week. *Treatment:* Chapter 7, all therapies; Chapter 8, Posture Therapies; Chapter 9, Reflexology; Chapter 10, Chiropractic, Osteopathy, Physical Therapy, Transcutaneous Electrical Nerve Stimulation; Chapter 14, Nonsteroidal Anti-inflammatory Drugs.

Multiple Sclerosis

Multiple sclerosis is an inflammatory disease of the central nervous system. Migraine-type headaches affect 27 percent of people with multiple sclerosis, and trigeminal neuralgia (see later in this chapter) occurs in up to 8 percent. Use of steroids in sudden, short-term flare-ups can be dramatically helpful. Research for prevention of multiple sclerosis has proved unfruitful thus far, although recent studies indicate that attention to diet, especially certain fatty acids, can produce positive results. *Treatment:* Seek conventional medical care. Elimination of wheat gluten, milk, and other foods known to cause allergic reactions may bring relief. Natural anti-inflammatories, especially essential fatty acids and vitamin C, may be helpful. See Chapter 11, The Healthiest Eating Plan, Elimination Diet Plan, and Omega-3 and Omega-6 Fatty Acids; see also Chapter 7, all therapies, and Chapter 10, Physical Therapy.

INFECTIONS

Headaches often accompany common viral conditions such as flu, the common cold, and mononucleosis, as well as serious infections such as viral meningitis, tuberculosis, and herpes zoster (shingles). Bacteria and other infectious organisms, such as *Pneumococcus* and *Salmonella,* also can cause headaches, as can rare diseases such as Lyme disease, typhoid, and malaria. Headaches can persist for weeks or months after an acute infection has gone away. If your headache lingers or is severe or unusual in any way, have a physician rule out the possibility of meningitis or other problem (see Meningitis, below). *Treatment:* Seek medical care. Immunity-enhancing herbs and food supplements can help fight the infection and provide pain relief; see the box entitled "Immune-System Boosters" in Chapter 11. See also Chapter 7, all therapies; Chapter 8, *Chi kung,* Yoga; Chapter 9, Oriental Massage, Reflexology.

Sinusitis

Sinusitis means "inflammation of the sinuses" and occurs when a bacterial or viral infection or some kind of irritant causes the membranes of one or more of the sinus cavities to become inflamed and exert pressure in the face and head. The result is often headache and nasal congestion as well as a runny nose. Cigarette and other smoking are a primary cause of sinusitis. Sinusitis also can be caused by an allergy to smoke, incense, animal hair, ragweed, or other airborne irritants. Actions that increase sinus pressure, such as coughing, bending over, and sneezing, usually make the pain worse. Frequently, sinus acupressure points on the face are tender to touch (see Chapter 9).

Chronic sinusitis occurs when the sinus cavities are blocked frequently or for several months at a time. In many chronic cases, a dental infection is the cause of sinusitis. Aggressive treatment of sinus infection and dental infection is recommended, as sinus passages are close to the brain and the infection has the potential to extend into that area.

Prevention and treatment: Your physician may take x-rays of your sinuses to determine if there are any deformities in the cranium or fluid in the sinus cavities. Most people have a "deviated septum"—asymmetrical nostrils—and this usually is not the cause of sinusitis. Regular use of nasal decongestants is generally discouraged, as they can cause side effects, such as rebound congestion and irritation of the nasal passage. They also should not be used by people with high blood pressure, irregular heartbeat, heart disease, or glaucoma. In P.M.'s experience, homeopathic nasal sprays are nearly 100 percent effective in eliminating allergy-related sinusitis. For more natural therapies, see Chapter 9: acupressure provides relief; acupuncture is frequently curative; also see Polarity Therapy. In Chapter 10, see Hydrotherapy. Avoidance of mucus-causing foods, such as dairy products, may be all that is needed to prevent recurrent sinusitis; see Chapter 11.

Inhalation of steam or application of hot compresses to the sinuses three to four times a day, 15 minutes each time, increases blood flow to the area and relieves pressure. Another effective therapy is nasal douching (see box on page 53).

Meningitis

Meningitis is a life-threatening central nervous system disease. In the majority of cases, it is caused by viral, bacterial, or fungal infection that has brought on inflammation of the meninges, the membrane around the brain and spinal cord. Only a lumbar puncture test can provide an accurate diagnosis. Meningitis is characterized by a severe headache, which can be anywhere in the head. It is accompanied by fever, stiff neck, nausea and vomiting, rash, joint pain, general malaise, and sensitivity to light; confusion, irritability, and coma also may occur. *Treatment:* Owing to its serious nature, immediate treatment is required; antibiotics may be curative, depending on the type of meningitis. To help deal with the stress associated with the disease, see Chapter 7.

Herpes Zoster (Shingles)

Herpes zoster is the return of the chicken pox virus most people think was destroyed after their bout with the disease as a child. However, the virus can lie dormant inside the nerve cell bodies near the spinal cord and brain. In about 10 percent of American adults, the virus is reactivated—either by stress or by unknown causes—and leaves the nerve cell body. The virus travels along

NASAL DOUCHING

Nasal douching is a therapy frequently prescribed by ear, nose, and throat specialists and is also a yoga practice that can relieve headache, inflammation, and other symptoms of sinusitis without irritation and drugs. Nasal douching involves use of a mild salt-water solution to rinse out mucus and clear the sinus passages of viruses and bacteria. This practice often makes people sputter and cough at first; proceed slowly.

Dissolve ¼ tsp. salt in 8 oz. warm water. Add ¼ tsp. goldenseal powder or colloidal silver to kill bacteria. Using more salt will draw water from the nasal membranes, and using less will cause the nasal cells to take up water. Both of these situations will irritate and cause burning or swelling. To use the solution, tilt your head forward and to the side and try one of the following:

- . . . Pour the solution into a saucer or your cupped hand and gently inhale the liquid through the upper nostril while you close the other with your finger; or

- . . . Gently squirt the liquid into the nostril using a bulb syringe; or

- . . . Slowly pour the solution into the nostrils from a small container with a spout, such as a Neti pot available through yoga supply dealers.

The solution will travel through one nostril into the other one, down your throat, or into the nasal sinuses, depending on your head position. To get the solution into all the nasal passages, it helps to roll your head around a bit. As you flush, blow your nose. Spit out any excess that goes into your mouth. Flush the nasal passages a few times or until the solution runs out clear. You can douche several times a day as needed.

the nerve to the skin supplied by that nerve and causes a painful rash of small fluid-filled blisters or red spots. These are often accompanied by headaches and fever. Frequently, pain occurs days before the rash appears. The risk of developing shingles is greatest for people who have a weakened immune system. Although the disease usually occurs in people older than 50 years of age, shingles appears to be affecting more younger people.

Shingles can infect the facial nerves, including the trigeminal nerve (see Trigeminal Neuralgia later in this chapter), and result in severe, sometimes persistent head pain. If the sight branch of the trigeminal nerve is affected, blindness can result. The rash and pain typically last 3 to 5 weeks. In some individuals, however, the pain persists after the rash is gone, while others experience pain without rash. This pain is difficult to treat regardless of the method; in most cases, however, both natural and conventional therapies can be effective. *Prevention and treatment:* See a doctor immediately if you notice the symptoms of herpes zoster mentioned above. Thymus extract, as well as certain dietary changes that affect acidity and amino acid balance and immune status, can decrease the pain and rash. For persistent pain, see Chapter 9, Acupuncture; Chapter 10, Transcutaneous Electrical Nerve Stimulation; Chapter 14, Antidepressants, Narcotic Analgesics, Capsaicin (Zostrix, among others).

INJURY

Head Trauma

Head injury—a concussion, a blow to the head, or a fall—commonly causes headache or pain at the injury site. If it is severe or does not clear up within a few hours, or if you have mental confusion, dizziness, or loss of consciousness, go to your hospital's emergency department immediately.

The brain is suspended in the skull and surrounded by fluid. When the head is hit, the brain tissue can be bruised, support structures can be stretched, and tiny tears and bleeding may occur. The resulting head pain is variable and may occur as pounding, pressing, aching, squeezing, burning, stabbing, or throbbing. It is usually, but not always, constant, and can involve any area of the head. The headache is typically made worse by coughing, jolting, moving the head, sneezing, bright lights or noise, alcohol consumption, physical exertion, or anxiety. *Treatment:* As a precaution, medical attention is recommended for head pain caused by trauma.

Whiplash Injury

After a whiplash injury, approximately 75 percent of people experience either daily (59 percent) or occasional headache (14 percent). These headaches are extremely variable; they can radiate from various muscles and other soft tissues in the neck, shoulders, and upper back and be felt in the face and head. *Treatment:* Suggested initial treatment includes gentle osteopathic or other hands-on therapy by an experienced specialist; see Chapter 10. Also see Chapter 7 for relaxation therapies; Chapter 9, acupuncture, acupressure, and therapeutic touch; and Chapter 13 for homeopathic muscle relaxants and anti-inflammatories such as arnica. Also, homeopathic agents injected into trigger points are as effective as steroid injections and do not have side effects. Application of heat to the head and neck provides relief. Also see Chapter 14, Antidepressants.

"PRESSURE" HEADACHE

"Pressure" headaches occur when pressure is placed on the brain, either by a tumor, clot, or lesion or by high blood pressure.

Transient Ischemic Attack

A transient ischemic attack (TIA) is a temporary loss of blood supply to the brain caused by a clot or lesion. Signs of this "small stroke" include temporary numbness, tingling, or weakness in an arm or leg or on one side of the face; temporary blindness; and difficulty with speech. If you experience these symptoms, see a physician immediately.

Approximately 25 percent of individuals who have a TIA experience a mild to moderate headache. The pain usually begins after the attack, although occasionally it happens before, and it can affect any part of the head, with most people having pain on the sides. Most of these headaches last about 2 hours; some linger for months. To accurately diagnose a TIA, physicians consider symptoms as well as the results of computed tomography (CT), magnetic resonance imagery (MRI), or other tests. *Treatment:* See Chapter 7, for relaxation therapies, after you have a diagnosis from your physician.

Brain Tumor

Head pain associated with brain tumors can appear in many forms and may resemble tension or vascular headaches. Headaches associated with brain tumor tend to become progressively worse as the tumor grows and are aggravated by straining, sneezing, coughing, bending the head forward, or any motion that increases pressure within the skull. The pain is frequently worse in the morning and is sometimes accompanied by nausea with or without vomiting. The pain may extend to any part of the head, depending on the location of the tumor. Other symptoms of brain tumor can include numbness or weakness in the arms and legs, double vision or blurring, and seizures that cannot be attributed to fever, an illness, or an accident. A definitive diagnosis of a brain tumor is made by MRI or CT. Not all brain tumors are cancerous; other growths can place pressure on delicate brain tissue and cause pain and neurologic changes. *Treatment:* Although surgical removal of the tumor is usually necessary, some of the stress and anxiety that accompany this condition can be reduced using the relaxation therapies in Chapter 7. Though lesser-known herbal agents are generally safe, it may be unwise, while you are under a surgeon's care, to experiment with them. Once you have been cleared of surgical or oncological care, you may wish to explore this option. Otherwise, manage your "alternative" remedies with a specialist who is trained in both conventional and other methods.

Hypertension

Headaches associated with high blood pressure can occur at any time of the day. Some people with high blood pressure who typically have a headache upon awakening take a blood-pressure pill and get pain relief. Others develop headaches when a rise in blood pressure is brought on by stress or poor diet, especially intake of too much salt or foods that cause an allergic reaction. *Prevention and treatment:* Life-style and dietary changes can often result in a significant decrease in blood pressure and thus reduce any head pain associated with it. See Chapters 7 and 8, all therapies; Chapter 9, Reflexology; Chapter 11, The Healthiest Eating Plan, B Vitamins, Magnesium and Calcium, Omega-3 and Omega-6 Fatty Acids; Chapter 12, Dong Quai, Valerian.

Benign Intracranial Hypertension

Also known as pseudotumor cerebri, benign intracranial hypertension (BIH) is characterized by increased pressure in the brain that occurs when there is too much spinal fluid inside the head and surrounding the brain. This can happen when the body makes too much spinal fluid or if the mechanism that absorbs excess fluid is defective. People with BIH typically have vision disturbances and migrainelike symptoms: nausea, pounding headache, vomiting, and hallucinations. Because sight is threatened, prompt medical attention is needed. To diagnose this condition, physicians typically determine what it is *not*—brain tumor or other brain lesion, intracranial infection, or hemorrhage, for example—and this determination is made by using CT, MRI, or lumbar puncture to examine the cerebrospinal fluid. Several different medications can cause BIH; see Table 6-1 in Chapter 6 to determine if you are taking a drug known to trigger BIH.

BIH occurs eight times more often among women than among men and is seen most often in young (age range, 20 to 44 years), overweight women who have menstrual irregularities. *Treatment:* After treatment for any visual loss has begun, diuretics are often given to relieve cerebrospinal fluid pressure; see Chapter 14.

NEUROLOGICAL CONDITIONS

The most common neurological disease that causes headache is cerebrovascular disease. Others include trigeminal neuralgia and epilepsy.

Cerebrovascular Disease

People who have a subarachnoid hemorrhage—bleeding into the brain usually caused by a ruptured or an abnormal blood vessel or veins in the brain—experience with it what many call "the worst headache of my life." The pain usually comes on rapidly, is severe, and typically lasts several days, although slow bleeding or rupture can occur without head pain. A "warning" headache may precede the onset of bleeding by 1 day to several months. The headache is often accompanied by nausea, vomiting, mild fever, stiff neck, hypersensitivity to light, dizziness, and an unstable walk. A recurring headache may indicate rebleeding. If you have a sudden intense headache, especially if you are older and have heart attack risk factors—high blood pressure, elevated blood lipid levels, being overweight, male gender, family history of heart attack, being a smoker—see your physician, who may schedule a CT scan or an angiogram in order to make a diagnosis if your symptoms are suggestive. *Treatment:* In addition to life-style changes (diet, smoking, alcohol), see Chapter 7 for relaxation therapies.

Trigeminal Neuralgia (Tic Douloureux)

Trigeminal neuralgia is a very painful condition that occurs when the trigeminal nerve, which runs down the side of the face, becomes inflamed (see Figure 5-1). This nerve supplies the face, teeth, mouth, and nasal cavity with feeling and the jaw and mouth muscles for processes such as chewing and talking. Trigeminal inflammation may be caused by pressure against the trigeminal nerve anywhere along its course, although it usually occurs at its root where it leaves the brain. Pressure may come from a nearby artery or veins or (rarely) a tumor. Inflammation also may be caused by a virus. Trigeminal neuralgia affects women more than men and is more common in people 40 years and older. The headache pain is stabbing, comes on suddenly, and usually lasts only a few moments, although it often repeats several times a day for days or weeks at a time. The pain is often triggered by chewing, talking, swallowing, or touching the gums or face. *Treatment:* Homeopathic injections or injections of lidocaine or steroids are erratically effective. Other options include acupuncture, antidepressants, and the antiseizure medication carbamazepine. Individuals who do not respond to medication may need to undergo surgery, although the pain may recur even after surgery.

Epilepsy

Approximately 50 percent of individuals with epilepsy have headaches after experiencing a seizure. The pain is usually throbbing, moderately intense, and lasts for several hours. *Treatment:* See Chapter 7, all therapies.

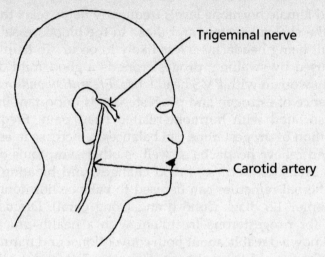

Figure 5-1
The trigeminal nerve in relation to the carotid artery.

HORMONE-RELATED HEADACHE

An imbalance of the female hormones estrogen and progester-one has been associated with migraines in women. Of women who have migraines, about 60 percent of the episodes are linked with the menstrual cycle and many are associated with the cycle exclusively. Headaches may be caused by the sudden decrease in estrogen levels that occurs in menopause or by water retention caused by an increase in estrogen during premenstrual syndrome (PMS).

There are several mechanisms that may cause PMS headache. The most common cause is an imbalance of female hormones. Estrogen influences salt retention, and high levels of salt lead to fluid retention, which causes swelling of tissue in the brain and thus headache. By the time menstruation begins about 14 days after ovulation, both estrogen and progesterone levels are at their lowest levels. Although some researchers believe that the low estrogen levels in the latter part of the menstrual cycle cause the blood vessels to expand and cause migraines, it is becoming clear that hormonal fluctuations affect the cells and likely trigger blood vessel changes. We do know that maintenance of regular, balanced female hormone levels frequently helps relax the muscles of the skeletal system and those in the blood vessels, with the result being headache is less likely to occur. To help relieve pain caused by swelling, progesterone is a good mild diuretic for many women with PMS headaches. *Prevention and treatment:* The balance of estrogen and progesterone is important in headache associated with hormone-related head pain. Frequently, the addition of progesterone can balance an increase in estrogen levels and relieve headache as well as other symptoms of PMS, such as breast tenderness, mood changes, and bloating, while several herbal remedies can be used to balance hormone levels (see Chapter 12: Black Cohosh and Dong Quai). Discuss your options for progesterone treatment with a health practitioner who is knowledgeable about both conventional and natural hormones. For natural therapies, see Chapters 7, 8, and 9, all therapies; Chapter 11, The Healthiest Eating Plan; Chapter 12, Black Cohosh, Dong Quai, White Willow; Chapter 13, pulsatilla.

Hormones also play a role in headache pain during other life situations:

- During the first trimester of pregnancy, some women experience worse headache pain than before they were pregnant and then become headache-free during the last two trimesters. Women who experience migraines associated with menstruation generally notice an improvement in the pain when they become pregnant. This appears to be due to the hormonal changes that occur during pregnancy.
- The prevalence of migraines tends to decrease with age, yet there is no consistency in how individual women respond to the decline in hormone levels that occurs at menopause. Some women's symptoms lessen on hormone replacement therapy (estrogen alone or with progesterone); others do not.
- Use of oral contraceptives containing estrogen and progestins can have various significant effects on occurrence of headache. Studies of oral contraceptive use and headache show that the hormones can initiate new headaches, aggravate existing headaches, trigger a woman's first migraine, increase the severity of headaches or migraines, or even decrease headache pain.

- Hormones can be adversely affected by stress, and head pain caused by water retention, muscle spasm, and other reasons—many as yet not well defined—can result from hormonal imbalance.

If you suspect a hormonal problem is contributing to your headaches, we recommend you seek a health-care provider who is familiar with hormone testing (see Appendix I).

OTHER MEDICAL CAUSES

Carotidynia

Carotidynia is a pain syndrome that affects one side of the head and neck. The main physical finding is tenderness when the carotid artery is touched (see Figure 5-1). The pain is usually throbbing, dull, and continuous and sometimes radiates to the cheek, ear, or eye. Difficulty swallowing, chewing, and moving the head toward the unaffected side are characteristic. The actual cause and frequency of carotidynia are unknown. Migraine is often associated with this condition. Some researchers believe that carotidynia is two or three times as common as cluster headaches. *Treatment:* See Chapter 14, Nonsteroidal Anti-inflammatory Drugs, Ergot Alkaloids, Beta-blockers, Calcium Channel Blockers, Antidepressants.

Chronic Fatigue Syndrome/Immune Deficiency Syndrome

Chronic fatigue syndrome/immune deficiency syndrome is an umbrella term that is used to include the many causes of this common syndrome. More than 90 percent of individuals with chronic fatigue syndrome experience headaches. The cause of the chronic fatigue may be the cause of the head pain, but this varies among individuals. The pain may be either tension or migrainelike and needs to be treated based on triggers and other influences.

Glaucoma

Glaucoma is an eye disease that can result in partial or total loss of vision. It appears in 2 percent of people older than 35. When the liquid inside the inner eye becomes blocked and cannot flow properly, the build-up of pressure causes damage to the optic nerve and can cause head pain.

Usually glaucoma appears as a low-grade, diffuse headache that lingers for years before vision loss is noted and glaucoma is diagnosed. Some patients report seeing haloes around lights.

In 10 percent of glaucoma, characteristics include severe eye pain that affects the entire head, blurred vision, extreme sensitivity to light, nausea, and vomiting. Recognition of this type of glaucoma, which appears most commonly among the elderly, may be diagnosed as a sudden first or worst attack of migraine. It requires immediate medical attention, as it can result in blindness within 3 to 5 days. *Prevention and treatment:* Have yearly eye examinations or a check for glaucoma if you are 50 years or older or if you have a personal or family history of the disease.

More than 90 percent of cases of headache pain do not have an underlying medical cause. To give you peace of mind—and allow you to receive immediate attention in the unlikely case that your headache does have a medical cause—we recommend you see your physician if you suspect your headache is associated with a medical condition. The sooner you have a diagnosis, the sooner you can explore natural therapies to help relieve your pain.

6

OTHER HEADACHE FACTORS:
FROM SEX TO ICE CREAM

As the headache wheel (see page 13) has shown us, there can be many factors besides stress or medical conditions that cause headaches. In this chapter, we look at headaches that are associated with specific influences, not related to named medical conditions, in these categories:

- *Diet/nutrition,* including food, beverages, food additives, and nutritional supplements
- *Environment,* such as toxic fumes or weather conditions
- *Drugs/medications,* both legal and recreational, and alcohol
- *Life style/physical stress,* such as overexercise, poor sleeping habits, and sex

These four areas cover a lot of territory, so we discuss the headaches that are reported most often in each one and how to prevent and treat them naturally.

To see if your headaches might be caused by one or more of these influences, answer the questions in the box on pp. 64–65.

COULD IT BE A HEADACHE WITHOUT A MEDICAL CAUSE?

Diet/Nutrition

Do you ever experience headache pain after eating any of the following?

- Hot dogs, bacon, ham, or sausage

- Fudge, coffee, or cola drinks

- Chinese food

- Ice cream or other very cold foods

- Foods or beverages that contain the artificial sweetener aspartame (NutraSweet)

Do you often miss meals or experience low blood sugar symptoms?

Have you had headache pain after starting a new vitamin program?

Environment

Are any of the following situations a part of your life?

- Exposure to toxic substances (for example, new carpeting, paint, new paneling, chemicals at work or at home, pesticide sprays)

- Sudden weather changes, perhaps due to traveling

- Exposure to increased or unusual lights or sounds

- Travel to high altitudes (above 8,000 feet)

- Confinement to unventilated or poorly ventilated room or building

Drugs/Medications

Do you use recreational drugs?

Have you started taking any medications, prescribed or over-the-counter?

Have you made any changes in dosage or frequency in current medications or stopped taking a particular drug?

Do you get head pain after drinking alcohol?

Life Style/Physical Stress/Posture

Are any of the following situations or activities a part of your life?

- Insufficient sleep or a change in sleeping patterns

- Smoking

- Travel over time zones

- Increase in or unusual amount of physical activity (for example, weekend athlete—sedentary all week and then run 5 miles on weekends)

- Sitting for extended periods of time at a desk or in a car, bus, train, or plane

- Standing for long periods of time

IF YOU THINK YOU HAVE A HEADACHE CAUSED BY OTHER FACTORS

Although many factors can contribute to a headache, recognition and management of the primary influences can be enough to bring significant relief. The rest of this chapter looks at various headaches that can arise from different common factors and offers some natural treatment options.

DIET-RELATED HEADACHES

Eight to 10 percent of all migraine headaches are triggered by foods, beverages, nutritional supplements, or the additives in these products. Some studies place the figure as high as 90 percent. In any case, many holistic practitioners agree that controlling dietary factors is second only to controlling stress in the successful management of headache and that good nutrition is key in the prevention and treatment of headache pain. Recommended nutritional guidelines are given in Chapter 11.

Very frequently, food has a role in headache pain, for a variety of reasons. You may be sensitive or allergic to a specific compound in a food, for example, or a food may affect your blood sugar level. In addition, some foods cause water retention or increase muscle tension; others promote constipation, which is a common cause of headache.

Not everyone is affected by the same foods, and some people may not respond one day and then react the next. Sometimes a single food is the sole trigger of a headache; usually a combination of substances, situations, or other factors precipitate head pain. If you eat a chocolate brownie while reading on Monday and don't get a headache but eat another brownie on Wednesday after you've had a fight with your kids and then you get a headache, it may be the combination of stress and chocolate that triggered the pain. If you had a glass of milk with that brownie, the milk, too, could be part of the cause.

Our genes may set us up to be susceptible to certain elements and conditions—say, chocolate and bright lights—that can trigger headache. According to Joel Saper, M.D., a clinical professor of medicine at Michigan State University, people either do or don't have the tendency to get food-related headache: "It is built in and it's genetic," he says. "What you eat can then influence that susceptibility, triggering headaches." Because food is a factor we can usually control, it is worthy of our sincere attention as a headache factor.

AVERSION, ALLERGY, OR INTOLERANCE?

The popular press leads us to believe that true food allergies can cause headache, yet in reality, the different food items that cause these allergies are frequently not investigated by practicing physicians. *Allergy* is a hypersensitivity to a food or other substance (called an allergen) that does not normally cause a reaction. In a true allergic reaction, the body's immune system is called into action. The body reacts to the allergen either immediately or over varying lengths of time by producing different types of antibodies. The number of antibodies the body needs to produce before a person reacts to a particular allergen varies. Immediate reactions include headache, asthma, hives, nausea, vomiting, swelling, rash, diarrhea, intestinal cramps, and life-threatening anaphylaxis. To determine which foods, if any, cause immediate hypersensitivity or acute food allergy, most physicians use a blood test or skin prick test to check for the immunoglobulin IgE. The most common types of headache caused by food, however, are the result of a longer-term immune reaction. To identify slow, or delayed, allergic reactions to food, your doctor must test for another immunoglobulin—IgG4. Several types of tests can identify IgG4, and some are more accurate than others. (See Appendix I, Environmental Medicine, for the names of laboratories that offer IgG4 testing.) Elimination diets and careful use of a food/symptom journal also can be used to identify food allergies.

Food aversion is a real phenomenon in which people have a subconscious connection between a food, either by smell or taste, and an emotional trauma from their past. With food aversion, the body may react with stomach distress and headache, among other symptoms.

Food intolerance is the common term for food reactions that are not associated with the immune system (that is, no antibodies are produced), yet the body is sensitive to the food and the result is headache pain. Several types of food intolerance headaches are explained below, including those caused by cold foods, nitrates and nitrites, monosodium glutamate (MSG), caffeine, alcohol, vitamins, and amines.

PREVENTION AND TREATMENT

For the diet-related headaches discussed under the headings below, the following general strategies are recommended.

- See the headache diary in Chapter 2 (page 18) and Elimination Diet Plan in Chapter 11 for help on identifying and treating food-related headache.
- Once you know or suspect which foods you are allergic or sensitive to, we recommend that you avoid them completely for as long as it takes for your body to "forget" to react; this may be 6 months to 2 years, especially in cases of true food allergy. Response to this method of dealing with food allergies and intolerance is highly individual. If you reintroduce offending foods before your body forgets them, you may react with a more severe headache than you had previously. In many cases, foods that once caused an allergic response can eventually be reintroduced into your diet in moderation, without causing problems, if you allow your body enough time to forget.
- Many methods are available to neutralize the effects of

food reactions, increase the body's ability to rid itself of the offending substances, and decrease inflammation. Vitamin C, the B vitamins, antioxidants, hormone balancing, adrenal support, homeopathics, and certain herbal remedies also can help to minimize food allergy symptoms. See Chapter 11, Nutritional Supplements as Treatment; Chapter 12, Fringe Tree, Milk Thistle, Tetterwort.

- As a general rule, relaxation therapies are helpful in food-related headache.

Ice-Cream Headaches

Consuming extremely cold foods such as ice cream or iced beverages can cause pain in the forehead, deep in the nose, in the temples, behind the cheeks, or occasionally in the ear. The pain is sudden, sharp, and strikes when the cold substance hits the palate. Fortunately, the headache usually lasts only 20 to 30 seconds. People with migraine are particularly susceptible to ice-cream headache.

To lessen the chance of cold foods causing headache, eat smaller, warmer bites. Keep them in the front of your mouth for several seconds until the roof of your mouth has a chance to cool down.

Monosodium Glutamate Headaches

MSG is a flavor enhancer that is added to food, especially in Chinese restaurants. A small bowl of wonton soup, about 200 ml, may have 3 g of MSG, which is enough to bring on symptoms in sensitive people. Within 20 to 25 minutes after eating food containing MSG, you may feel a bandlike pressure around your forehead and pressure or throbbing over the temples. Flushing, a pressing pain in the chest, dizziness, tightness of the face, and abdominal cramps also are common.

MSG appears in foods under several aliases, including hydrolyzed vegetable protein (HVP), hydrolyzed plant protein (HPP), and "flavoring," "natural flavor," and kombu extract. It is most commonly used in soups and sauces, diet foods, salad dressings and mayonnaise, processed and frozen foods, potato chips, and dry roasted nuts. Read food labels!

Caffeine Headaches

Caffeine presents two faces to headache sufferers: on one, a cup of coffee can relieve migraine pain; on the other, the same amount can set your head pounding. People who are sensitive to caffeine should avoid all products that contain it, including coffee, colas, tea, chocolate, and over-the-counter and prescription medications given for headache.

Roger believed caffeine was causing his daily headaches, so one day, he just stopped drinking his usual three to four cups a day. Instead of feeling better, however, the headaches got worse. What happened? Caffeine is a drug—the single most common addictive drug in the United States—and Roger experienced caffeine withdrawal. To prevent withdrawal headache, a gradual decrease in consumption of coffee or other caffeine products is recommended. A good program is to taper slowly over 3 days for every cup you drink per day. Thus, it takes 1 month to wean off of 10 cups a day.

For some people, caffeine causes heart rhythm changes or bladder or prostate problems. Some physicians recommend that these individuals quit "cold turkey" and suffer through a few days of withdrawal symptoms—nausea, anxiety, fatigue, and depression—rather than continue drinking caffeine. To calm your nerves while you are withdrawing from caffeine, take supplements of B vitamins, vitamin C, calcium, and magnesium; see Chapter 11.

Nitrate/Nitrite Headaches

Meats cured with sodium nitrate/nitrite, such as hot dogs, sausage, bologna, bacon, and salami, trigger headaches in people who cannot tolerate this food additive. The headache usually lasts several hours and is sometimes accompanied by facial flushing. Researchers are not certain how these additives cause headaches, although one theory is that they cause the blood vessels to dilate, resulting in throbbing head pain. Tylenol is commonly prescribed for this type of headache.

Aspartame (NutraSweet) Headaches

The artificial sweetener aspartame has been linked to headaches—and especially migraines—in many people. Although study results conflict, it is generally agreed that some people are particularly susceptible to this additive and should restrict consumption or avoid it completely.

Amine Headaches

Many natural substances are toxic when taken in large amounts. Foods rich in amines (protein building blocks) can cause headache in some individuals. Tyramine is believed to be the biggest culprit in provoking migraine. It triggers the release of a substance called norepinephrine, which causes the blood vessels in the brain to constrict. When the norepinephrine is depleted, the blood vessels expand, and the result is headache. Tyramine is found in citrus fruits, aged and hard cheeses, herring, liver, nuts, cured and processed meats, some yeast products, figs, raisins, broad beans, and chocolate.

Chocolate is one of the few foods that contains phenylethylamine, another amine that causes the blood vessels in the head to dilate and cause migraine-type pain. In fact, one study showed that people who have migraines have significantly lower levels of a platelet enzyme that breaks down these amines. If you suspect amines are causing your headache pain, use the headache diary (Chapter 2, page 18) or the elimination diet (Chapter 11) to help you make a more positive identification.

Hypoglycemia

Abnormally low blood sugar levels—hypoglycemia—brought on by missing a meal, dieting, or fasting, or too much insulin in the body, causes headache by several mechanisms. Thus, people who are hypoglycemic are much more likely to experience migraine than those who are not. Adherence to a frequent, regular meal schedule of small meals or snacks between meals usually prevents these headaches. Avoid sugary foods and eat frequent meals that consist of a balance of complex carbohydrates, protein, oils, and vegetables. See Chapter 11, The Healthiest Eating Plan, and Chapter 12, Dong Quai.

Gastrointestinal Problems

Sometimes headaches are associated with the way the body processes food. For example, you may get constipation and a headache if you don't get enough exercise or enough fiber in your diet. The latter can be corrected by taking $^1/_2$ tsp. of psyllium husks or seeds once a day in 1 cup of water, followed by a second cup of water. Large doses of vitamin C (2,000 mg every few hours) and 1 tbsp. of flax oil, if necessary, can bring prompt relief. In addition to improving your diet, you can drink peppermint tea to relieve the bowel distension. Headache associated with the digestive tract also can come from bowel gas in the body, overeating, or food allergies, among other causes of gut-related headache.

To help prevent and treat headache associated with gastrointestinal problems, see Chapter 11, The Healthiest Eating Plan; Chapter 12, Catnip and Devil's Claw (for gastrointestinal discomfort); and Chapter 13, nux vomica (for constipation).

NUTRITIONAL FACTORS

Elevated or deficient levels of certain vitamins and minerals in the body may be associated with an increased risk for development of headaches or migraines. The nutritional elements that are most commonly associated with head pain are discussed below. If you think your diet may have an imbalance of any of these vitamins or minerals, see Chapter 11 under Nutritional Supplements as Treatment for the foods that contain these nutrients and the Recommended Daily Allowance (RDA) values.

Vitamin A

Believing that if a little is good, a lot must be better, some people take large doses of vitamin A or eat foods that have high levels of the vitamin because it is noted for helping eyesight. As a fat-soluble element, however, vitamin A is stored in tissue and fat and can build up to toxic levels. Although individuals vary greatly in their tolerance for vitamin A, dosages greater than 60,000 IU (international units) cause headache. The good news is that the pain begins to disappear 1 or 2 days after you reduce your intake. Other toxic effects of vitamin A, including harm to the fetus, are not apparent until the damage is done. It is much safer to balance your vitamin A intake with beta-carotene supplementation.

B Vitamins

Deficiencies of vitamin B_6, B_{12}, and folic acid are associated with headaches. Poor diet and use of birth control pills can result in B vitamin deficiency. Vitamin B_6 is important in many biochemical processes, including magnesium utilization and protein metabolism. A deficiency in this vitamin appears as muscle weakness, nervousness, and irritability. People with a deficiency of vitamin B_{12} typically have fatigue and possibly headaches, memory loss, changes in personality or mood, tingling in the hands or feet, and muscle weakness in the legs or arms. If you suspect a vitamin B_{12} deficiency, ask your doctor to run a blood test. Some people need a B_{12} level of 800 pg/ml to get relief.

Sometimes the symptoms of B_{12} deficiency actually indicate low levels of another B vitamin—folic acid. Americans typically consume about 50 percent of the folic acid they need. Combine that statistic with another fact—that aspirin intake can produce a folic acid deficiency—and you may be treating a headache with a substance that is contributing to it. Besides headache, folic acid deficiency appears as fatigue, forgetfulness, anemia, irritability, and anorexia.

Choline and Chromium

Blood levels of choline are low in people with headache, and pain symptoms improve when choline levels increase. This may be due to hypoglycemia, which improves with choline intake. There also may be a link between low choline levels and cluster headaches. Chromium, too, plays a role in headache caused by low blood sugar.

Copper

Copper is important as a cofactor for blood vessels to constrict and contract. It appears that migraine headaches may occur more often when blood levels of copper are low. Symptoms of copper deficiency include fatigue, paleness, skin sores, and swelling.

Iron

The average adult body contains between $1/2$ and 1 tsp. iron, yet let that amount slip just a little low and you may have a headache. Other symptoms of iron deficiency include dizziness, weight loss, anemia, weakness, constipation, and decreased appetite. Iron deficiency affects women more than men because of blood loss during menstruation, and it is especially evident in pregnant women and teen-age girls.

Magnesium

One of magnesium's key functions is to maintain the tone of the blood vessels. Several studies show a substantial link between low magnesium levels and both migraine and tension headache. Deficiency of this mineral appears as fatigue, premenstrual syndrome (PMS), anorexia, irritability, cravings for chocolate, insomnia, and muscle cramps.

DRUG-INDUCED REBOUND HEADACHES

Headaches are a potential side effect of many drugs, some of which are actually prescribed to *relieve* headaches. Such headaches are called *drug-induced rebound headache* and can be debilitating. The head pain caused by drugs taken for headache and other various ailments and diseases varies in severity, location, and type (see Table 6-1).

A drug-induced rebound headache is chronic. More than 80 percent of Americans who have chronic daily headache overuse analgesics; for simple analgesics, this means more than 1,000 mg aspirin or acetaminophen daily for 5 or more days a week, for example. Sometimes it is difficult to determine if overuse leads to chronic headaches because it looks like the opposite to the sufferer. Characteristics of drug-induced headache include the following:

- Daily or almost daily use of headache medication, yet headache is not relieved
- Early-morning awakenings because of headache
- Abdominal cramps, diarrhea, nausea, sleeplessness, restlessness, nervousness, irritability, and an increase in intensity of the headache—all withdrawal symptoms—after suddenly stopping daily headache medication

After the initial period of withdrawal (usually 5 to 7 days) from the culprit drug is over, headache severity and frequency gradually decrease and sleep and well-being improve. Occasionally, medication withdrawal requires hospitalization.

Drug-induced rebound headache is considered to be a tension headache. For more information and treatment strategies, see Chapter 3, Chronic Daily Headache and How to Prevent and Treat Tension Headache.

TABLE 6-1.
Drugs with Headache as a Possible Side Effect

Generic Name	Treatment Indication*	Trade Name(s)
Acetaminophen	C	Tylenol
Acetaminophen, aspirin, and caffeine	C	Excedrin
Aspirin and caffeine	C	Anacin
Atenolol	H, M	Tenormin
Benzphetamine	HY	Didrex
Betamethasone	BIH	Celestone
Captopril	H	Capoten
Cimetidine	H, M	Tagamet
Clonidine hydrochloride	HY with rapid withdrawal of Catapres	
Cortisone	BIH	Cortone
Dexamethasone	BIH	Decadron, Dalalone
Dextroamphetamine	HY	Dexedrine
Diclofenac	H, M	Voltaren
Ergotamine tartrate	C	Cafergot
Estrogen-containing oral contraceptives	M, C	Brevicon, Demulen, Enovid, Lo/Ovral, Norinyl, Ortho-Novum, Ovcon, Ovral, Triphasil
Fenfluramine	HY	Pondimin
Fluoxetine	H	Prozac
Flunisolide	H	AeroBid Inhaler
Griseofulvin	H	Fulvicin, Grisactin, Gris-PEG
Hydrocodone bitartrate with acetaminophen	C	Vicodin
Hydrocortisone	BIH	Cortef, Hydrocortone
Hydromorphone	C	Dilaudid
Indomethacin	H, M	Indocin

Interferon	H	Intron A, Retrovir IV, Roferon-A
Isocarboxazid	HY	Marplan
Isosorbide dinitrate	H	Dilatrate-SR, Isordil, Sorbitrate
Lithium	HY	Cibalith-S, Eskalith, Lithane, Lithobid
Mazindol	HY	Sanorex
Meperidine	C	Demerol
Methylphenidate	HY	Ritalin
Methylprednisolone	BIH	Medrol, Depo-Medrol
Metoprolol	H	Lopressor
Morphine	C	
Nalidixic acid	HY	NegGram
Nifedipine	H, M	Adalat, Procardia
Nitroglycerin	H	Minitran, Nitro-Bid, Nitrolingual, Nitrodisc, Nitro-Dur, Nitrogard, Nitrong, Nitrostat
Oxycodone with acetaminophen	C	Percocet, Tylox
Pemoline	HY	Cylert
Phenelzine	HY	Nardil
Phenmetrazine	HY	Preludin
Phenylpropanolamine	HY	Allerest, Comtrex, Contact, Dimetapp, Sinarest, Tavist-D
Phenytoin	HY	Dilantin
Piroxicam	H	Feldene
Pramethasone	BIH	Haldrone
Prednisolone	BIH	Delta-Cortef, Hydeltrasol
Prednisone	BIH	Deltasone
Propoxyphene	C	Darvon
Ranitidine	H, M	Zantac
Terazosin	H	Hytrin
Tetracycline	HY	Achromycin, Panmycin, Robitet, Sumycin
Tranylcypromine	HY	Parnate
Triamcinolone	BIH	Aristocort, Nasacort
Trimethoprim-sulfamethoxazole	H	Bactrim, Septra

---

*H = headache, tension type; M = migraine; HY = hypertension that may result in headache; C = chronic daily headache; BIH = benign intracranial hypertension and severe headache.
(Compiled from *Monthly Prescribing Reference,* 11, January 1995, and Solomon, Seymour. *The Headache Book,* Yonkers, NY: Consumer Reports Books, 1991, p. 23.)

HEADACHES FROM RECREATIONAL DRUGS AND ALCOHOL

Smoking marijuana reportedly can both trigger and relieve headache. Headache caused by marijuana tends to be in the front of the head and can be treated as tension headache (see Chapter 3).

Cocaine causes blood vessels to constrict and is associated with migraine-type pain and symptoms. Withdrawal from cocaine also can cause headaches. High doses of vitamin C are helpful in treatment of withdrawal symptoms from narcotics.

Alcohol causes the blood vessels to dilate, and when consumed in excess or by those who have a low tolerance for alcohol, it can cause nausea and vomiting in addition to head pain. Everyone has a different tolerance level for alcohol, and some varieties cause headaches in certain people and not in others. This difference may be due to a sensitivity to the additives in alcohol, such as esters, acids, tannins, and aldehydes. Red wine and bourbon have the highest number of these additives; vodka, the lowest. That does not mean, however, that vodka cannot trigger a headache.

To prevent alcohol-related headache, avoid alcohol completely or drink very little. Alternately eat while you drink and have a snack high in fructose (honey, jelly, fruit juice) before you go to bed. Alcohol-related dehydration can cause headaches, so drink a lot of water with alcohol. Also, take an antioxidant combination that contains at least 2,000 mg of vitamin C. For treatment of alcohol-induced nausea, see Chapter 12, Chamomile, Hops, Peppermint; and Chapter 13, nux vomica and pulsatilla.

ENVIRONMENT-RELATED HEADACHES

As with food-related headaches, the best way to prevent head pain related to environmental factors is to avoid the things that initiate the pain. However, it is not always easy or feasible to do so. If you work in an automobile repair shop, for example, or you travel a great deal, you may have routine exposure to elements or situations that cause headaches. Below are some environment-related headache types and how to deal with them. In all cases, the relaxation therapies in Chapter 7 are helpful.

High Altitudes

Headache caused by being at high altitudes is known as acute mountain sickness or altitude sickness and is characterized by a throbbing or pounding pain in the front or back of the head. The pain begins between 6 and 96 hours after you reach high altitude, typically 10,000 feet and higher. Coughing, sneezing, exertion, straining, sleep, and reclining all make the pain worse.

To prevent altitude sickness, avoid alcohol while at high altitudes. Drinking cold fluids reportedly is helpful. Acclimate yourself to each increase in elevation: a general guideline is to ascend no faster than 800 to 1,000 feet per day once you are above 8,000 feet. Avoid overexertion and get plenty of rest. Also see Chapter 14, Diuretics, for relief.

Chemical Fumes and Environmental Irritants

Both short-term and long-term exposure to chemical fumes or environmental irritants (see box on page 78) can cause headache. You may be breathing these fumes at work (in an art studio or paint factory, for example) or at home (perhaps your furnace is malfunctioning or you have a new carpet that is giving off fumes). Cleaners, petroleum products, compounds found in building materials—even perfumes and incense—can cause headache pain in sensitive people. The pain is usually described as pressure, although it may be throbbing at times. Short-term exposure to toxic fumes also can cause dizziness, blurred vision, yawning, tremors, hypertension, nausea, palpitations, and various other symptoms. Chronic exposure usually causes a dull headache in the front of the head and is accompanied by chest pains, nervousness, difficulty in concentrating, and vertigo. Confusion, stupor, or delirium also can occur with long-term exposure. Changes in mental state and the types of other problems vary, depending on which gas or fumes you are exposed to.

To prevent this type of headache, make sure ventilation systems are working properly, and wear a face mask if necessary. Discuss toxic exposure situations with your employee advocate at the workplace or your landlord, as appropriate. Find a physician who specializes in environmental medicine and who is familiar with tests and treatments for this growing problem (see Appendix I).

CHEMICAL AND ENVIRONMENTAL TOXINS KNOWN TO CAUSE HEADACHE AND ALLERGIC REACTIONS

- Aluminum dust
- Automobile exhaust
- Chromium and cobalt in cement
- Coal fumes
- Dyes
- Factory smoke
- Fluorocarbons
- Formalin
- Glues (in carpet, flooring, wallboard, furniture, etc.)
- Grain dusts
- Insecticides
- Motor oil
- Organophosphates
- Paints
- Perfumes, deodorizers
- Platinum salts and acids
- Polyvinylchloride
- Solvents
- Wood dusts

Seasonal and Perennial Allergies

Seasonal allergies are an allergic reaction to pollen—weed, tree, and grass—during specific seasons of the year and are often referred to as hay fever, although neither hay nor fever is usually involved in this condition. Perennial allergies are reactions to agents people are exposed to year round, the most common of which are house dust, house dust mites, mold spores, and pet hair. Typical symptoms of perennial and seasonal allergy include nasal congestion; watery eyes, runny nose; itching of the nose, throat, roof of the mouth, and inside of the ears; headache; and sneezing spells.

Avoidance of the irritant is the best medicine. Other helpful measures include thorough cleaning of the carpets and upholstery and wearing a face mask. Some herbal remedies are effective; see Chapter 12, Ephedra.

Weather

Some people can predict changes in the weather by the onset of migraines, while others can predict their migraines by the arrival of bad weather. A switch from low- to high-pressure systems is the most common headache trigger. Warm, humid weather is worse than cold and dry, although both types of weather can initiate head pain.

Noise

Exposure to short- or long-term high levels of noise can trigger headaches. Loud music and noisy machinery are two common sources. If you cannot avoid noisy situations, use earplugs. To prevent future ear sensitivity, wear earplugs during loud concerts and other noisy events, when riding in small airplanes, and when near or using large power tools, loud engines, or machines.

Odors

People who get migraines are especially susceptible to odors, and many say their headaches get worse when they are exposed to certain smells. The offending odors may be those most people find quite pleasant, such as perfume and baking bread, yet they trigger pain in a growing number of people who otherwise do not have headaches. Tobacco smoke, perfume, and room deodorizers can trigger headache in many people, regardless of their tendency to get migraines.

Bright Lights

Sunlight and overhead fluorescent lights are the primary sources of headache pain in this category. If you are exposed to the glare of sunlight reflected from water, sand, or snow or you drive into the rising or setting sun, the muscles around the eye can become tense and the blood vessels may dilate. Glare from overhead lights can cause a similar response.

You may avoid headaches from bright lights if you wear sunglasses outdoors and photosensitive glasses indoors where overhead lights are a problem. For headaches caused by overexposure to the sun, see Chapter 13, nux vomica and euphrasia.

LIFE STYLE/PHYSICAL STRESS-RELATED HEADACHES

Sex Headaches

Sex headache is not the "not tonight—I have a headache" type of head pain but the headache that begins during sexual activity and typically peaks at orgasm. It occurs in men four times more often than in women and more often in people who get migraines. Most people who experience headache during sexual activity initially have a dull pain that grows into a very intense throbbing or "explosive" pain; some have a dull or tension-type headache. Either type may last for several minutes or hours.

The increase in muscle tension, blood pressure, heart rate, and blood vessel dilation that occurs during sexual activity is a possible cause of head pain. Because the explosive nature of this headache type is shared by conditions such as stroke, meningitis, sinusitis, glaucoma, and encephalitis, it is best to be examined by your physician if you experience this type of pain.

To ward off this headache, relax and breathe deeply either before or when you first feel the headache building. Let your shoulders drop and open yourself to feel your emotions. This may be all you need to resolve your pain (see Chapter 7). This is an opportunity for you and your partner to use and enjoy the relaxation and bodywork therapies in Chapters 7, 9, and 10. Herbal and homeopathic preparations are also good for headache prevention. Also, avoid intercourse positions that increase pressure to the head or restrict circulation. For a medical approach, see Chapter 14, ergotamine tartrate and Beta-Blockers.

Cough and Exertion Headaches

Sometimes physical exertion causes a sharp pain in the head that lasts for seconds to several minutes. This can be brought on by exercise, such as running or weight lifting, or by coughing, sneezing, laughing, stooping over, or straining on the toilet. Cough and exertion headache may be caused by a brief increase in pressure in the head that occurs during these activities, although muscle strain is the more common cause. More men than women experience these headaches, and they occur more often in people who have migraines.

Headache associated with flu and cough is common. A virus can irritate the lining of the brain and spinal cord as well as the neck and head muscles. Such head pain can last for days to weeks.

Because cough and exertion headaches generally last only a short time, treatment usually is not an issue. Relaxation therapies (see Chapter 7) are effective, especially if coughing or sneezing is persistent. To prevent headache associated with exercise, the first step is to relax and recondition the neck muscles. Herbal and homeopathic treatments are helpful. For a conventional approach, see Chapter 14, Nonsteroidal Anti-inflammatory Drugs. Codeine is useful as a cough suppressant and pain reliever.

Eyestrain

If you work at a computer screen, read for extended periods of time, or work with detailed material, you may experience excessive contraction of the muscles in and around the eyes. This eyestrain often leads to headaches. To prevent eyestrain, take a five-minute break from the activity at least once every hour. Spend the time practicing some of the natural therapies offered in this book. Also try the following quick treatments: (1) cup your eyes with your hands, imagine you are looking at black velvet, and focus on that blackness for several minutes; (2) hang your head down between your legs and breathe deeply; then slowly sit up and do chair twists by turning first to one side and then the other; (3) periodically look away from your work and gaze into the distance. You should have your eyes checked professionally. Also see Chapter 13, euphrasia.

Sleep

The brain houses a biological clock that regulates functions such as appetite changes, waking, and sleeping. When you disturb that clock by getting too much, too little, or irregular sleep, the result can be headaches. The cause of sleep disturbances is not always obvious and may be a combination of factors, such as stress, workaholism, too much caffeine, depression, a side effect of medications you are taking, or poor sleep habits. For relief, see Chapters 7 and 8, all therapies; Chapter 9, Oriental Massage, Polarity Therapy, Reflexology. For stress reduction, see Chapter 13, Scullcap, Hops, and Valerian. Homeopathic remedies are usually helpful. **Note:** Headaches are only one symptom of insomnia, which can have a significant effect on your family and work life. If you take sleeping pills or antidepressants, do so under the care of a physician.

Swim-Goggle/Tight Hairdo Headaches

Head pain can result from continued pressure against nerves in the head from wearing a tight hat or swim goggles. Remove the hat or goggles periodically to relieve the pressure and massage your temples. After you take the hat or goggles off completely, use *chi kung* (Chapter 8); acupressure, Oriental massage, reflexology, or therapeutic touch (Chapter 9); or myotherapy (Chapter 10). Head pain caused by tight ponytails or cornrows responds to the same therapies except myotherapy.

There are dozens of factors in everyday life, unrelated to medical conditions, that can cause headache pain. This chapter has highlighted some of the most common factors in the hope they can help you identify which ones may play a part in your head pain.

PART II

NATURAL MEDICINE FOR HEADACHE RELIEF AND PREVENTION

Welcome to the relief and prevention portion of this book. As you use this section, remember that the aim of natural medicine is to bring all aspects of a person into balance. You may be lucky and find one herb or one exercise that relieves your headache pain. More likely, however, you will need to make changes in several areas of your life for the relief to be long lasting. As a general rule, good nutrition, adequate exercise, sufficient sleep, stress reduction, and spiritual and emotional fulfillment are all necessary for balance and well-being.

The following chapters contain natural therapies that you can use to self-treat or have a friend perform for you, and those that require a professional to perform. Both types of treatments are clearly indicated in their respective sections. Generally, self-treatment is safe; however, it may be wise to have a complete physical examination by a physician to rule out the slight possibility that your headaches are caused by a medical condition that needs to be treated, especially if you have medical problems. Ideally, seek a physician who respects the power of the life-style changes and natural therapies you have chosen and who understands the potential side effects and drug interactions of any prescription or nondrug remedies you are currently taking.

If, after you have been examined by your general practitioner, you try self-treatment and you are not happy with the results, you may want to contact a natural medicine practitioner to assist you. All of the natural therapies in this book contain self-treatment techniques for you to try, except for a few therapies, such as craniosacral therapy and osteopathic, for which professional treatment is required. In these latter cases, we explain what a typical treatment session involves.

Many patients with headaches who make changes in their life style, such as improving their diet, managing stress, or starting an exercise program, find that their weight, blood pressure, and cholesterol levels move toward or become normal and they can reduce or stop the amount of medications they take. Have your blood pressure and other health indicators monitored regularly and your medicine and dosages adjusted by your doctor.

As you seek out practitioners of the various disciplines in this section, you will find that many of them are skilled in more than one therapy. Most holistic therapies lend themselves very readily to working in combination. An acupressure therapist may also be adept at reflexology and therapeutic touch or a craniosacral therapist may also do massage therapy. As an individual looking for pain relief, you can benefit greatly from such multitalented professionals. Unless your practitioner is monitoring the effect of a single remedy, such as homeopathic therapy, the advantage of combining several natural therapies—for example, meditation, yoga, and acupuncture—is that this usually increases the effect of your pain relief.

Regardless of the practitioner you choose, it is most important that she or he be caring, knowledgeable, well connected and respected in the community, and know when to make referrals. Good luck and good health.

7

RELAXATION
TECHNIQUES

Stress is the single most significant influence contributing to headache pain. It is very likely that whatever headache pain you have, it can be decreased, if not resolved, with conscientious use of the skills presented in this chapter.

When your brain senses stress, it puts out nervous signals and releases hormones that affect every cell in your body. This "stress response," or fight-or-flight response, originally described by Hans Selye in the 1950s, is exactly the opposite of what happens when you relax. Everyone has a unique reaction to the stress response, based on their genetics, experience, and physical environments, all of which create their attitude and response to stress.

In the late 1960s, Herbert Benson, M.D., of the Harvard Medical School, described what he called the "relaxation response" as "an inborn set of physiological changes that offset those of the fight-or-flight response . . . [and these] changes are coordinated [and] occur in an integrated fashion." This response can be elicited in several ways, such as meditation, yoga, prayer, deep breathing, visualization, hypnosis, and progressive muscle relaxation. Many individuals combine several techniques or switch according to what works best for them. Subsequent research has confirmed Dr. Benson's finding, and he is convinced it "can help in the treatment of many medical problems; in some cases, it can eliminate them entirely . . . [and] to the extent that any disorder is caused or made worse by stress, the relaxation response is useful," although he is quick to emphasize that it never should be substituted for conventional medical care. It is, however, a "scientifically proven treatment that is totally compatible with other approaches of modern medicine."

The beneficial effects of relaxation techniques frequently go beyond elimination of habitual headaches. Deep breathing may improve your patience and flexibility with others. Visualizations may increase your capacity to give and receive good feelings. Meditation may enhance your spiritual connectedness. Choose the relaxation therapies that attract you most and that have the "side effects" you desire.

In this chapter, we review some of the most popular, effective, and interesting ways to relieve stress and reduce, eliminate, or prevent head pain. We begin slightly out of alphabetical order with breathing, because proper breathing is basic to all life and using it will support whatever therapy you choose. It is followed by biofeedback, hypnosis, meditation, progressive relaxation, self-talk, and visualization.

BREATHING THERAPY

Breathing is something we take for granted unless we have trouble because of congestion, injury, illness, or exertion. Yet when you focus on your breath, you can use it to help relieve or eliminate any kind of pain. According to Eastern tradition, energy is understood in both practical as well as religious terms. In India, the energy of life is called *prana*, which is derived from the syllables *pra*, which means "first unit," and *na*, which means energy. "All the diverse forms of this universe are sustained by the energy of *prana*," says Swami Rama, who showed, under scientific scrutiny, the ability of the mind to control physical functions thought to be beyond our control. "One who has learned to control *prana* has learned to control all the energies of this universe . . . [and] to control his body and his mind."

To understand how to breathe properly, watch how babies do it. Babies instinctively do diaphragmatic breathing: the entire torso rises and falls. This utilizes the strongest breathing muscles and is the powerful way to breathe. It is used in yoga (see Chapter 8) and is the breathing technique referred to frequently in this book. There are many variations on deep breathing for relaxation and other benefits.

Before we discuss breathing therapy for headache pain, here is a basic breathing exercise that, with practice, can quickly put you into a state of deep relaxation. "The single most effective relaxation technique I know is conscious regulation of breath," says Andrew Weil, M.D., one of the world's leading authorities on health and medical therapies, in *Natural Health, Natural Medicine*. He recommends the breathing exercise in the box below for everyone. It is the perfect prelude to the rest of this book . . . and the rest of your life.

You can do the exercise in the box below in any position. If you are seated, keep your back straight. Practice this breathing technique at least twice a day and whenever you feel stressed or the need to focus your thoughts and think clearer.

BREATHING EXERCISE

1. Place the tip of your tongue against the ridge behind and above the upper front teeth. Keep it there throughout the entire exericse.

2. Exhale completely through your mouth, making a "whoosh" sound.

3. Inhale deeply and quietly through your nose to the count of 4 (with mouth closed).

4. Hold your breath for a count of 7.

5. Exhale through your mouth to a count of 8, making a sound.

6. Repeat steps 3, 4, and 5 for a total of four breaths.

BREATHING TO RELIEVE HEADACHE PAIN

To practice breathing, get comfortable—either lie down or sit in a cozy chair. Loosen tight clothing. Place your hands over your rib cage and abdomen and feel the movement as you breathe. Now, take a deep breath and breathe into your belly. Feel the breath begin at the belly button and carry the abdomen and chest easily with it. The breath expands the upper lungs and reaches down until you can feel the pressure of it in your pelvis. Let the air enter each cell, without strain. Hold the breath for a moment of deeper relaxation, then exhale fully from the belly button area first, with the chest and pelvis both following without effort. The emphasis is on a long, slow, and complete exhalation that allows your abdomen to fall toward your spine. Do not squeeze or contract. Enjoy the blissful rest after the exhalation when you are empty and at peace. Watch your rhythm, and let each inhalation and exhalation last longer and longer, becoming easier and easier. Focus on the air that goes into your abdomen and how it feels as it comes out.

GUIDED BREATHING MEDITATION

The box on pp. 91–93 is a guided breathing meditation that a friend can read to you or, preferably, you or someone else can tape it so you can reuse it. Speak very, very slowly and clearly. This narrative is written for you to breathe in pace with the words. Some people record soft meditative music in the background of the tape.

Choose a time and place you can be undisturbed for about 10 minutes. Get into a comfortable position in which you are as pain free as possible. If you are lying face up and can do so, rest your right hand on your belly and your left hand on your chest to better feel the rise and fall with each breath. Shift your hands or your body at any time to remain comfortable. If any stray thoughts float into your mind, gently postpone them until later. Let your awareness be completely on your breathing.

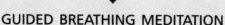

GUIDED BREATHING MEDITATION

Breathe in slowly through your nose. Breathe out with lips slightly parted, the tip of your tongue in the groove behind your front teeth at the floor of your mouth. Breathe in evenly and fully. Breathe out evenly and fully. Feel the moment of stillness after you exhale.

Breathe in to a steady count of 7. Breathe out to a count of 12, tapering to a peaceful, empty pause. This will guide your cycle to its maximum of relaxation and to a healthy balance of oxygen intake and carbon dioxide release.

Breathe in, and your breath gently pouches out your belly and then expands easily into your chest. . . . Feel the out breath release the air without effort. . . . Feel the in breath expand your lower lungs, expanding your torso like a balloon. . . . Breathe out, and the balloon passively empties from the belly and chest together. . . . The in breath fills you up and out in all directions. . . . The out breath releases tension from every part of your body. . . . See yourself expanding with the in breath, relaxing your muscles even more as you breathe out. . . . Inhale relaxation: feel it deeply in all of your muscles; relax your mind. . . . Exhale your tension, again, from all of your muscles, from your mind. . . .

As you feel more focused, you begin to feel the subtle physical expansion of the in breath. . . . Breathing in gently stretches the ligaments surrounding the spine and opens the spaces between the back bones. Breathing out releases the tension of these ligaments and settles the bones in line with gravity. . . . The in breath gently stretches the fascia that surrounds and connects your organs and muscles. . . . The out breath releases tension throughout your body and mind. . . .

As you breathe in and out, focus on the spot four finger breadths below your navel in the center of your lower abdomen. . . . As you breathe deeply into this warm place, feel your pelvis open like a flower in all directions. . . . As you breathe out, your pelvic bones, like petals, subtly fold in and the pelvis settles down around this spot, your energy "furnace." . . . On the in breath, the pelvis tucks in and expands and lengthens your lower back, straightening the arch and tipping your bottom forward. . . . The out breath releases the gentle stretch of the lower back muscles into its subtle elastic arch. . . .

Feel the warmth increase from your center and open up your pelvis with the breath in. . . . Feel the warmth spread up and out through your entire body as you breathe out. . . . Feel the warmth spread into your buttocks and flow down your legs as you breathe in. . . . Feel your legs release and melt, heavy and warm as you breathe out. . . . The opening out of the pelvis during inspiration very subtly opens the legs out at the hips. . . . The folding in of the pelvis during expiration very subtly rotates the legs in at the hips as they fall with gravity. . . .

Feel your lower spine open and round out with the in breath. . . . Feel this area of the spine settle with the out breath. . . . The midtorso rounds out like a swelling, flexible barrel as you fill with air and relaxation. . . . The entire midportion of your body falls gently inwards as you passively let the air out. . . .

Feel your chest walls open out on both sides and increase your width from front to back. . . . Feel the relief as the chest walls return to a position of release during the out breath. . . . Feel the incoming air lift the upper chest, expanding your front, back, and both sides. . . . Feel the outgoing breath carry with it any emotions you experience with the movement. . . . The spine and back muscles are gently stretched on each in breath and released by gravity while you breathe out.

Let the opening in breath flow into your collarbone area and shoulder girdle. . . . Let the settling out breath place the bones and muscles of your upper torso in a position of balance and effortlessness. . . . Again, the inflow of awareness expands in all directions and lightens the walls of your torso like a spaceship lifting off, then settling back down. . . . Feel your throat subtly opened by the inflowing air. Feel the back of your neck lengthen and settle as you release your breath between your parted lips. Feel the breath carry awareness into and fill your throat. . . . Ever so slightly, your neck lengthens, front and back. . . . As you exhale, again feel the back of the neck stretch subtly. . . . After your breath is fully exhaled, relax into the peace of the moment between the exhalation and your next in breath. . . .

Feel your neck muscles relax, and when you are completely full of air, relax even more and let the air release slowly, passively, from your belly, chest, and upper airways. . . . The in breath lifts the shoulder up and out so that your arms and hands very subtly rotate outward. . . . The out breath releases the shoulder girdle to its most comfortable and effort-free position by gravity. . . .

Feel the in breath wash through the muscles of your head, expanding the back of the skull ever so slightly. . . . Feel the out breath massage the muscles of your face and jaw as it releases slightly forward. . . . Feel a subtle expansion of the back and top of your head as you breathe in fully. . . . Feel a release of mental and emotional tension as you relax fully. . . .

Complete your breathing exercise with a unifying breath felt throughout your body and mind. Feel your inspiration to its fullest. . . . Open and be invigorated. Feel your expiration to its fullest. . . . Let go and be released. Carry this peace and awareness with you as you move about and interact in life.

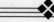

HOW DOES BREATHING ALLEVIATE HEADACHES?

A breathing exercise like the one in the box on page 89 eliminates head pain because it results in deep relaxation and releases muscle tension. Like other relaxation techniques, deep breathing has many benefits, including a strengthening effect on the immune system. According to many Eastern disciplines, full, deep breathing is essential to health. Deep breathing is recommended as part of your daily routine; practice it while you sit in your car at a red light, wait in line, or whenever you feel tense.

BIOFEEDBACK

It may be hard to believe that you can control the width of your blood vessels by consciously focusing on them. Yet that is just one thing biofeedback training can help you do. Biofeedback allows you to control functions in your body that are usually involuntary, such as temperature, heart rate, and blood pressure, to relieve tension and headache pain. To try this painless therapy, all you need is patience, practice, and something to let you know you're on the right track, such as a temperature gauge or a device that displays your blood pressure or pulse rate. Biofeedback is effective: overall, 75 percent of people with severe chronic headaches say they experience some relief from this therapy. Permanent relief results from ongoing practice.

BIOFEEDBACK FOR HEADACHE PAIN

Biofeedback is effective for tension headaches, migraines, and headaches caused by high blood pressure. It is often used along with other relaxation therapies—especially meditation and visualization—and it complements drug therapy to the point that you probably will need less medication as you practice it.

Initially, you will need the help of someone trained in biofeedback to help you learn the techniques. Many large cities have a center or teaching facility that provides biofeedback, and some physicians offer it. (See Appendix I for help in finding a location.) Biofeedback is ideal for people who want objective evidence of their success and like electronic gadgets. Biofeedback is frequently reimbursed by insurance companies and is available in many pain clinics.

HOW DOES BIOFEEDBACK WORK?

The biofeedback equipment makes you aware of your body's own signals and abilities to control pain. While your body's responses are being monitored, you can actually see or hear indications of when and how your body is sending these signals to you. Your increased awareness of these signals can help you learn to make the mental and physical adjustments needed to decrease or eliminate the headache. Many people report that simply feeling less helpless about their pain is beneficial. In *Mind/Body Medicine,* one research team reports that at least 50 percent of patients notice a 50 to 80 percent improvement. The number of visits you need will depend on the severity of your headache pain and how much you practice at home.

Tension Headache

During a biofeedback session for tension headache, you will have monitoring devices called electrodes, like those used in an electrocardiogram, attached to the skin of your head and possibly your neck. These electromyograph sensors send signals back to a monitoring device. The monitor has a rising and falling needle on a meter, audible beeps, or other indicators that show when your muscles are relaxed and when they are tense. Techniques vary: commonly, you are shown how to concentrate alternately on relaxing and tensing your muscles as the monitor keeps you apprised of your progress. With practice, you can learn to keep your muscles relaxed and prevent or control your pain without using the machine. Other biofeedback monitors track heart rate, blood pressure, breathing rate, and hand temperature (see below) for signals that show if you are relaxed.

Migraine

Migraine sufferers often have cold hands and feet because of poor circulation. To relieve the pain of migraines, biofeedback specialists monitor skin temperature using "thermal biofeedback." This technique helps you to relax the vessels, receive more blood flow into your hands and feet, and thus relieve the pressure in the blood vessels in your head.

To do this, a temperature gauge is attached to your finger or toe while you visualize your hands or feet becoming warmer and warmer. Use whatever image works for you: perhaps it's sitting in front of a roaring fireplace, lying on a tropical beach, or imagining the physical effect of the vessels in your hands opening up to allow the blood to flow more freely there. Typically, you'll see a significant change in the temperature on the gauge after four or five visits. Once you master the technique with the machinery, you need to practice without the machinery to get lasting benefit. This takes about 15 minutes a day. Some people can warm their hands in just seconds after they have practiced for a while.

Biofeedback is effective in migraines with and without aura. Some individuals with aura, however, find biofeedback to be most successful if they practice temperature feedback when the first signs of the aura appear. An analysis of 23 studies of the effectiveness of thermal biofeedback in patients with migraine with aura shows a 52 percent improvement in headache pain; another analysis of 22 studies shows a 49 percent improvement in patients who combine thermal biofeedback and autogenic training (see Hypnosis, below).

Other Headaches

Biofeedback is effective in relieving headache pain in which stress and tension are factors, including headache associated with high blood pressure. To gain the most benefit from biofeedback for headache associated with high blood pressure, it is best to practice biofeedback daily.

HYPNOSIS

Hypnosis, either induced by another person or by oneself, is an altered state of awareness in which individuals are highly compliant, relaxed, and susceptible to suggestions and commands that reach the unconscious directly. It is a way to communicate directly with the unconscious. While in a hypnotic state, people's attention can be focused on things of which they otherwise may not be aware. Have you ever driven to a familiar location, such as to your job or to the store, and once you arrived you couldn't remember how you got there? That is an example of a mild hypnotic state.

Not everyone is susceptible to hypnotic suggestion: about 20 percent of people are very susceptible, while another 20 percent may not respond at all. The rest respond in varying degrees. A common misconception is that people will do things that are against their principles or beliefs while hypnotized. This is not true. When you are in a hypnotic state and are given a suggestion, the conscious part of you maintains its perception of and control over acceptable behavior, so you will never do anything while in a hypnotic trance without the permission of your conscious self.

HOW DOES HYPNOSIS WORK?

Hypnosis allows you to sharply focus your attention on healing. There are many different techniques you can use once the mind is focused: distraction, reprogramming to less painful ways of thinking, substituting another physical response to stress, processing causes of stress to find alternatives in your life, uncovering old emotions, among others. Many people who have learned self-hypnosis say it is well worth the effort, and studies have shown self-hypnosis to be effective in controlling migraine pain in both children and adults. Generally, most adults can learn to control their headache pain within two months if they practice the techniques daily.

HYPNOSIS FOR HEADACHE

It is best to go to a licensed hypnotherapist to either learn self-hypnosis or to be hypnotized. (See Appendix I for help in finding hypnotherapists; see Appendix II for where to find self-hypnosis tapes.) One technique a hypnotherapist may use to empower you to deal with your headache pain and then adjust the way it feels to you is explained below:

> The sensations you are feeling could be interpreted as painful, but you are going to experience them in another, more positive way. You can choose how you would like them to feel. Perhaps you want them to be cool or warm, tingling or itchy. Now, when you feel these sensations, you will have the power to feel them in the way you have chosen.

This approach does not address the cause of the pain, but it can help individuals with severe headaches to better cope with their pain and to decrease their fear of it, thus making it more manageable and bearable.

Another effective coping technique for severe headaches is called "symptom substitution." The hypnotherapist will suggest that you move your pain to another place in your body. Although this does not eliminate the pain, it "tricks" your nervous system into presenting the pain somewhere else. This approach can be very helpful, especially when you feel a migraine coming on, because it allows you to significantly reduce the pain's incapacitating power and to go on with your daily activities. Pain "sent" to your foot, for example, typically will not be associated with the mind-numbing pain and nausea that often accompany migraine pain. Symptom substitution demonstrates your innate ability to control the quality, quantity, and location of your pain responses. The most effective and permanent hypnotic techniques allow you to identify the habit or psychological cause of your pain and then to readjust your mental or physical reactions.

Fred always got a headache when he heard repeated tapping noises, like typing or raindrops on a roof. In a hypnotic session he recalled the first time this occurred—during a traumatic incident in his boyhood, an onlooker had been drumming her fingers on a table. Once he separated the painful memory from the noise to which it was previously associated, Fred had no more headache.

SELF-HYPNOSIS FOR HEADACHE: AUTOGENIC TRAINING

Many people are trained by a hypnotherapist to perform self-hypnosis, as it allows them to manage their pain on demand. One form of self-hypnosis is autogenic training, which was developed by Dr. Johannes Schultz in 1929. The goal of autogenic

AUTOGENIC HYPNOSIS PROCEDURE

- Prepare by doing deep breathing and becoming fully relaxed. As you breathe, repeat silently the phrase *I am at peace* until you reach a state of relaxation.

- Once you feel relaxed, repeat silently, *My right arm is heavy.* Repeat it several times while concentrating on your right arm. Observe how your right arm feels and notice any emotions or feelings that arise as you focus on your arm. There is no right or wrong way to feel; simply feel.

- Repeat silently, *My left arm is heavy.* Again, repeat it several times while concentrating on your left arm and observe any emotions or feelings.

- Do the same procedure for each of the following phrases:

    My right leg is heavy.
    My left leg is heavy.
    My arms and legs are heavy and warm.
    Heartbeat calm and regular.
    Breathing calm and regular.
    My center is warm.
    My forehead is cool.
    My neck and shoulders are heavy.
    I am _____ (give a personal affirmation, such as *I am at peace with myself*).

Ideally, this series should be done twice a day, 20 minutes each time. This simple technique can relieve or reduce headache pain, as it reduces muscular tension, regulates blood and energy flow, and helps you to relax completely.

CAN HYPNOSIS WORK FOR YOU?

Are these statements true about you? If so, chances are good that hypnosis will work for you.

- *I have a good imagination.* This includes all your senses. Although most people have a vivid imagination, some don't believe they do, and it is the *belief* that is important in hypnosis.

- *I want to take personal responsibility for my health.* When you take drugs to mask pain, you hand over control to the medication. With self-hypnosis, you take back the reins. This requires commitment to learn the technique.

- *I know exactly what I want out of self-hypnosis.* This is usually easy if you have headache—you want no pain! Elimination of pain may be your goal, but it is good to have others, too. For example: you don't want to lose time at work or school; you don't want to cancel social engagements; you don't want to spoil your vacation or holidays.

- *I am willing to dedicate the time it takes to learn self-hypnosis.* There are no self-hypnosis pills; it usually requires weeks, and sometimes months, of daily practice.

- *I want to know myself better, and I am willing to change and let go of old thought patterns.*

training is "I am at peace," and this state can be reached by silently repeating different exercises, or phrases, while concentrating on the body part that corresponds to the phrase.

Autogenic training can be done in a group or individually. You can learn the technique from a certified instructor or follow a self-help book on autogenics. To experience how this technique is used, try the procedure in the box on page 98 in a quiet, comfortable place where you won't be disturbed for 20 minutes.

MEDITATION

Meditation is not one but hundreds of different techniques that have a common purpose: the conscious attempt to clear the mind or still the "chattering monkey," the conscious part of the mind that is always busy with details, words, and thoughts about how the body will react in any situation. Once the "chattering" is stilled, the psyche and spirit are free to expand into new regions of consciousness. Meditation offers the opportunity to be freed of responses you make because of habit, such as tensing your neck and shoulder muscles whenever you are stuck in traffic or clenching your jaw when your kids fight. These responses, which cause muscle tension, blood vessel contraction, and ultimately headache pain, can be eliminated with meditation. (See Sources and Suggested Readings for books on different types of meditation and Appendix II for meditation tapes.)

HOW DOES MEDITATION WORK?

During meditation, the body enters a state of peace: natural relaxation chemicals increase, heart rate and breathing rate decrease, and muscle tension dissolves. Brain waves settle to slower, more regular patterns, such as alpha—the waves the brain usually puts out when, for example, someone stares, mesmerized by a campfire—versus their usual active beta state.

Psychologically, meditation allows you to "step back" from your thoughts, habits, and experiences. Once the mind is uncluttered and open, stress is reduced, muscle tension is released, and your thinking becomes clearer and more focused. Spiritually, meditation speaks to our deepest needs for connectedness and inner peace.

MEDITATION FOR HEADACHE

Meditation is an excellent way to relieve stress and achieve a state of overall physical and emotional relaxation. It can help prevent headaches and reduce or eliminate them once they have begun. To achieve these goals, we strongly recommend that you practice meditation daily; even 5 minutes can make a difference. You may make rapid progress if you meditate 20 minutes twice a day. Many people who meditate in the morning find they can start their day with a calm, focused foundation and that everything then seems to go much more easily. The following basic guidelines are for almost any type of meditation you select.

- Choose a room or space where you will not be disturbed and where you feel safe and at ease. You can sit on a chair, on a pillow on the floor, or wherever you are comfortable. Some people like to set out candles, precious items, flowers, or incense. Make the meditation space your special place.
- Begin by calming your mind. Deep breathing is a good way to do this. Use the breathing exercise given in the box on page 89. Teachers of many yogic disciplines recommend these tips for the best effect:

1. Sit upright so your spine is straight.
2. Relax your jaw and curl your tongue upward so the tip points to the top of your head.
3. Focus your eyes, with lids closed, upward to the top of your head.
4. Touch your fingers or hands in a closed circuit or touch them to your knees or feet to keep the energy flow contained.

- Choose a meditative focus. This can be anything you want; examples follow below.
- Let stray thoughts drift through your mind. This happens to everyone. Just allow them to float away like a feather in the wind and then return to your meditative focus.
- When you are finished meditating, remain quiet with your eyes closed for a few minutes and watch how this state infuses into your "waking" world.

Here are some general meditative focuses for you to consider. One is the *mantra* or sound meditation, in which you use a word or syllable to help induce or deepen your concentration. Choose whatever has special meaning for you and makes you feel peaceful and secure. Some people repeat words or phrases like *love, peace, harmony,* or *I am calm* or *I am light.* Others repeat parts of a prayer or a syllable like *om.*

Repeat your mantra aloud to yourself, saying it more and more softly until it is a whisper. Listen to it in your mind. You can close your eyes or keep them open, whatever is comfortable for you. Mantra meditation consists simply of sitting quietly in your special place and hearing your mantra in your mind. You can slow it down, make it get louder or softer, raise or lower the pitch. It doesn't matter; it is your mantra. Meditate for 15 or 20 minutes or whatever is comfortable for you and then gently return to full awareness of your surroundings.

A simple mantra, used with the breath, involves slowly taking a single deep breath and saying the word *in* to yourself as you inhale and *out* as you exhale. After that single deep breath, do not try to control your breathing. Every time you inhale and exhale, say the word *in* or *out* to yourself. Concentrate solely on repeating the words. Draw them out so they take up all your meditation: "innnnn" and "ouuuuuut." If your mind wanders, that's okay. Simply return to your words. When you feel ready, gently return and sit quietly.

Another technique is to focus on an object or place. Choose a simple natural object: a flower, rock, piece of wood, an acorn, leaf, or a space 3 to 6 feet ahead of you, even on the other side of a wall. Whatever you choose to focus on can be real or imaginary. If real, place the object three or four feet in front of you at or near eye level. Sit comfortably and allow your eyes to rest on the object, but do not *try* to focus or not to focus on it—just rest your gaze upon it easily. When your eyes wander, let them return to the object gently. Allow the object to remain in your field of vision for a comfortable amount of time—5 or 10 seconds for most people—and then let your eyes wander. Return your attention to the object whenever you are ready; you will "know" when the time is right for you. Every time you rest your eyes on the object, allow yourself to look at it innocently for 5 or 10 seconds and then let your eyes wander again. Continue this for about 5 minutes. Then close your eyes for 1 or 2 minutes and sit quietly.

A meditation technique derived from the Vipassana tradition, called *mindfulness*, teaches people to be fully present in every moment. The idea of mindfulness is to experience your surroundings with all of the senses with neutral acceptance, almost as if you were observing your life as you live it. A tool you can use to help you feel your pain without becoming overwhelmed by it is called *scanning*, in which you feel the pain in increments and with patience instead of as a whole, totally encompassing experience. If you are open to what you may learn emotionally about your pain, your awareness of it can shift the pain from a physical to an emotional level. You may even sense the pain as tingling or warmth. When you use breathing techniques and relax, the pain can shift and sometimes disappear completely.

To practice scanning, read the box below completely and then set aside at least an hour to practice, alone and in quiet.

There are also yogic and Taoist systems of meditation that teach your mind's eye to watch the energy flow along specific channels, or meridians. Some of these systems teach different flows for different healing purposes and are best learned from masters of the technique. (See Sources and Suggested Readings.)

HOW TO SCAN

Begin in a relaxed position, with eyes closed. Define your pain as a physical object with texture, color, temperature, smell. It can be anything: a rubber ball, a block of wood, a granite boulder, a blazing star. Imagine where it sits in your body and how it feels emotionally. Define its edges. Are they sharp? blurry? always changing? How do they change? You may give names or metaphors to help you define the symbol of this pain. Once you have a clear picture of the symbol or "thing," focus your mind at the top of it. Imagine that the center of your consciousness is sitting directly on top. Let your body feel what that is like; experience fully what the top view feels like. Breathe deeply. Take in just what you can, with an open, loving attitude. When you are ready, imagine there is a thin, central line that goes through the object. You will enter the object and sink down from the top toward the center of the thing, following this line. Don't try to see the sides, front, or back of the thing, just the thin central line. Slowly make your way to the bottom. This may take you a half hour or more. Once you reach the bottom, slowly rise again through the center to the top. Breathe easily and experience everything fully and without preconceptions or judgments. Once at the top, shift your awareness to the front of the thing and enter it. Feel along a fine line from front to back. Once at the back, turn around and come forward. That may be enough for you, depending on the time it takes and the emotional intensity you experience. You may be ready to move on to something else because the headache is gone! You may want to talk to someone about your experience, write about it in a journal, or draw a picture of it.

PROGRESSIVE RELAXATION

Progressive relaxation is an excellent technique if you are new to body-relaxation exercises because it draws your attention to each area systematically. Each muscle contraction you perform automatically brings relief of tension when you release the contraction.

This exercise is best done while lying on your back on a firm, comfortable surface such as an exercise mat or a thick blanket. A large recliner chair that supports your neck and head also can be used. Wear comfortable clothing and no shoes.

Progressive relaxation is taught by instructors from many different disciplines and often is a part of exercise and yoga classes. Self-help tapes also are available (see Appendix II).

PROGRESSIVE MUSCLE RELAXATION EXERCISE

Close your eyes and place your arms by your sides. Starting with your feet, tighten up the muscles in your toes and legs. Tense your arms, clench your fists and jaw, contract your stomach, and tighten your buttocks. Concentrate on how each body part feels when it is tense.

Take a deep breath through your nose, hold it for 3 to 5 seconds, and then release it slowly through your mouth as you release the tension in all of your muscles.

Now you will focus on individual muscle groups and tense and relax them individually while you keep the rest of your body relaxed. For each group, you will do the following: tense up the muscles; hold the tension for 5 to 10 seconds while you focus on how the tension feels; take a deep breath, hold it for 3 to 5 seconds, and then as you exhale through your mouth, release all the tension in those muscles.

Begin with your hands. Make tight fists. Feel the tension throughout your hands and arms. Relax and let the tension go. Press your arms down against the surface they are resting on. Hold the tension and then release it. Let your arms and hands go limp.

Shrug your shoulders toward your head and hold them there. When you release them, feel the tension drain away. Wrinkle your forehead. Hold it and then relax. Clench your jaw and hold your teeth together. Hold and then release. Open your mouth as wide as you can. When you release the tension, let your mouth hang open and then let your lips touch gently. Close your eyes tightly and then let them relax, still closed. Concentrate on how your face feels now that it is relaxed.

Take a deep breath and let the air fill your lungs. Hold it and feel the tension in your chest. Squeeze your shoulder blades together as you inhale. Exhale slowly and relax your chest. Tighten your stomach muscles, then relax. Arch your back, then let it fall gently toward the surface you are lying on as you exhale. Notice how the upper part of your body feels relaxed and calm.

Tighten your buttocks and hips. Press your heels and legs against the surface you are resting upon, hold it, and then relax. Focus on your toes as you curl them under. Feel the tension in your feet, hold, and then release your toes and the tension. Bend up your toes toward your kneecaps, hold, and then release.

Now start at your head and notice how soft your face feels, how relaxed your shoulders, arms, stomach, chest, hips, and legs feel. Spend a few moments to enjoy this relaxed feeling. When you are ready to get up, sit up slowly. Stand when you feel ready.

VISUALIZATION AND GUIDED IMAGERY

We all daydream from time to time, but we usually do not concentrate fully on the scene or image. In visualization, you allow a scene or other image to enter your mind's eye and then totally focus your attention on it. Although "visualization" implies the use of sight only, it is most powerful when you also imagine the sounds, smells, textures, and tastes that are associated with it. You can then use the visualization to relax and ease or eliminate headache pain.

You can learn visualization from self-help books or tapes, or you may take a class or private instruction. Once you have an image or scene in your mind's eye, you can use it with guided imagery, a technique in which you picture yourself in your scene and take a mental "trip" through it. Some people use guided imagery as part of their treatment for serious diseases, such as cancer and AIDS, and create whatever healing pictures in their mind they believe will eliminate or reduce their disease and pain. You can do the same thing for your head pain.

HOW DOES VISUALIZATION WORK?

Visual, auditory, and tactile (touch) imagery are produced in the cerebral cortex, the thinking and language center of the brain. Using a technique called positron emission tomography (PET), which maps brain activity, it has been shown that the cerebral cortex is equally activated whether people actually experience something or if they just create a vivid image in their mind. Thus, when we vividly visualize a scene or situation, the brain processes it as reality. The brain registers the picture and sends messages to the other bodily systems, including the autonomic nervous system, which regulates temperature, blood pressure, and heart rate. The body enters a state of peace: the brain's natural relaxation neurochemicals increase while heart rate and breathing rate decrease. As stress melts away, muscle tension decreases and so does pain. The more calming, joyful, and refreshing the sensual images are that you bring into your mind, the more effective the session will be. If you visualize sitting in front of a roaring fire in a winter cabin, for example, also visualize the snow outside. Smell in your mind's nose the aroma of pine trees or hot cocoa and hear the sound of crackling wood.

VISUALIZATION AND GUIDED IMAGERY FOR HEADACHE

Suggestions on how to use visualization for headache come from people who have used it successfully. Popular images include gardens, sanctuaries, and deserted beaches. Choose a scene that signifies peace and relaxation for you and hold the image in your mind's eye. Then you may choose to take a guided imagery "tour" like the one explained below. In guided imagery, you elaborate on the scene you have in your mind and create a story or situation that helps you relieve stress and pain.

For example, Natalie, a 29-year-old social worker who has frequent headaches, visualizes an enormous rose garden. She pictures herself touching the soft petals and smelling the wonderful aromas. Then she meets "a wise old mentor" whom she trusts completely. The mentor can be anyone—real or imaginary—such as an ancestor, a fairy godmother, or a friend. Natalie's mentor was an image of herself in perfect health: clearheaded and calm, with no headache.

Natalie begins a dialogue with the wise one using a series of "yes"-or-"no"-type questions, such as "Is this headache associated with stress?" and "Will you help me discover a better way to handle it?" As Natalie allows her childlike trust and imagination to emerge, she recognizes her desires as well as her wisdom and common sense and uses them to discover solutions to her stress.

The box below contains another type of guided imagery narrative commonly used by people with pain. This narrative allows you to travel into your body and, with your mind, give each part of your body what it needs to heal. You may want to read it aloud and tape it so you can reuse it. If so, pause 3 to 5 seconds at each ellipsis. Set aside about 15 to 20 minutes to complete your journey. Prepare by finding a quiet, comfortable spot where you won't be disturbed. Do the breathing exercise described in the box on page 89 to help you focus and clear your mind.

When you tap into your imagination and internal strength, you can learn to heal your own headache pain. This chapter has explained ways you can use the power of your mind to get such relief.

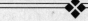

GUIDED IMAGERY NARRATIVE

Your mind is becoming clearer and clearer with every breath you take. . . . Every time you inhale, your mind becomes lighter . . . every time you exhale, your mind becomes lighter. Somewhere deep inside you, there is a light. Welcome it as you get ready to meet your headache pain. . . .

In your mind's eye, see the muscles in your neck and shoulders. . . . Find any tight areas, from the back of your head, down your neck, to your back and shoulders. . . . As you picture these taut muscles, send your breath into the back of your head, into your neck, into your shoulders . . . breathe into the area that is tight and feel as the tightness loosens. . . . See and feel your muscles gently against your neck, against your shoulders . . . imagine the tension flowing away from them as they lie there softly. . . .

Breathe into the feeling of looseness . . . feel the blood flow easily into your neck and shoulders and wash away the tension and stress. . . . Imagine the texture of the muscles in your neck and shoulders . . . feel how smooth they are . . . feel their warmth. . . . Feel each of the muscles in your mind's eye . . . imagine they are loose and free of tension. . . .

Picture the blood vessels in your forehead, in your scalp, in your brain . . . imagine you can touch the muscles in those blood vessels. . . . Feel if they are tight . . . feel their tension. . . . Imagine that they are getting supple as you touch them . . . picture the blood vessels opening up and letting the blood flow through freely. . . . Feel the blood course unhurriedly through your body . . . through your arms, your legs, your hands, your feet. . . . Feel your body become warmer as the blood moves through the blood vessels. . . . Imagine the tension gently lifting away from your head and out your fingers and toes . . . see it leave your body . . . feel the lightness. . . . Hear your breath become more faint.

Another type of visualization allows you to take a vacation from your pain and stress. Imagine you are in your favorite spot. See the colors . . . smell the air . . . feel the sun or the wind on your skin . . . fully experience all the scene offers you.

Breathe into the peace and calm of your surroundings. Experience the sensual pleasures of the scene as long as you can and invite the relaxed feeling to stay with you when you return to your worldly tasks.

Here is a quick way to adjust your discomfort level. In your mind's eye, imagine a thermometer on a wall. Picture the contents of the vial a bright red or a dark blue or black. As you focus on the cause of your pain or stress, notice how the fluid rises. Then let your tension go, and watch the fluid go down.

Now, scan your head, your neck, your shoulders . . . notice how the pain level has changed. . . . Breathe into the changes . . . praise yourself for allowing those changes to happen.

8

MOVEMENT THERAPY

Our bodies consist of a wonderful collection of muscles, bones, ligaments, joints, tendons, and fascia (membrane that covers, supports, and separates the muscles) that allows us incredible movement: to stand and dance, jog and swim, curl up and stretch. We want to keep these structures healthy because they are an integral part of our overall health. When muscles are tensed or stretched or pulled, wherever they are in the body, they can have a direct or indirect effect on causing or contributing to headache pain.

The most common cause of muscle tension headaches are contractions of the neck and shoulder muscles, which are a direct reaction to stress. When muscles are habitually shortened, they can stay tight and cause headache pain in several ways. Not only are the nerves to the scalp pinched; blood vessels, ligaments, tendons, and joint structures are compressed and can refer pain. A major form of referred pain is compressed muscles, which form trigger points, as discussed in Chapter 10.

In this chapter, we introduce several movement therapies to relieve headache pain: *chi kung* (a form of *tai chi*), yoga, and balance movements. This latter method consists of a series of movements developed by one of the authors (P. M.) for use with headache patients. They are designed to relax, lengthen, balance, and strengthen the muscles, particularly those in the neck and shoulders, which will help ease or eliminate your headaches, whether they are caused directly by muscle tension or not. These movements are best learned from a teacher or with videotapes (see Appendix II); therefore, this chapter presents only the high-lights and a summary of balance movements, as well as a few movements so you can "sample" them.

Other movement therapies, including the Feldenkrais Method and the Alexander Technique, focus on posture and can also help relieve headache pain. These two approaches are de-scribed in the latter part of this chapter.

CHI KUNG/TAI CHI

Chi kung, also called *chi gung*, is a form of *tai chi*, an ancient Chinese discipline that requires those who practice it to combine physical movement with deep concentration. This allows people to directly control their bioenergy flow and achieve relaxation, muscle tension relief, and relief from headache as well as other causes of pain. Although it appears to be primarily a physical movement, it is based on the philosophy that thoughts are inter-nal movements and that bioenergy follows thought. The more you practice *chi kung*, the more you perceive the energy move-ment, which many people describe as clear sensations of tin-gling, warmth, or gentle diffuse electricity that moves through them.

The closest Western translation of *chi kung* is "energy cultiva-tion" or "practice." If you are looking for a quick fix for your tension headache, *chi kung* is not your answer. If, however, you want an overall, long-lasting remedy for imbalance and head-ache pain, the slow, progressive nature of *chi kung* may provide it for you. Those who practice *chi kung* typically enjoy better overall health, a sense of balance, peace, relaxation, and greater emotional stability.

HOW DOES *CHI KUNG* WORK?

In Chinese philosophy, bioenergy, like life itself, is a continuous flow of change, much like the flow of a river—steady in its movement but also flexible when it encounters obstacles. The movements that make up *chi kung* stimulate the flow of bioenergy. As you concentrate on your physical movements, you also feel energy as it moves through your body. The combination of your physical movements and mental awareness promotes your energy to flow through blockages caused by physical and emotional tension. As you continue to practice day after day, your body will become stronger and more flexible. Your posture will improve, you will learn to relax, and tension and headache pain will drain away.

Some people report that their body seems much more receptive to other treatments once they take up *chi kung*. This makes *chi kung* an excellent addition to any other therapy you may be using.

CHI KUNG FOR HEADACHE

Chi kung consists of dozens of movements and variations of each one. The exercises are done slowly and in succession. Most are not strenuous and are done while you stand. In the box on page 113, we explain one of these movements. Although you can practice *chi kung* from a book, it is best to start with classes or get lessons from a master so you can see and appreciate the flow of the movements firsthand and have your posture and breathing corrected.

When performing *chi kung*, do not strain. Practice deep breathing and maintain good posture. This is essential to allow the free flow of *chi*. If you are at risk for stroke, have vessel disease, or have had neck surgery or a fractured cervical spine, consult your doctor about the safety of extending your neck (see "Read This First" box on page 118).

There are many *chi kung* movements that do not involve extension of the neck.

The ancient practice of *chi kung* is gaining in popularity. More and more people find that it is an excellent way to control headache pain, reduce muscle tension and stress, and attain a sense of overall well-being.

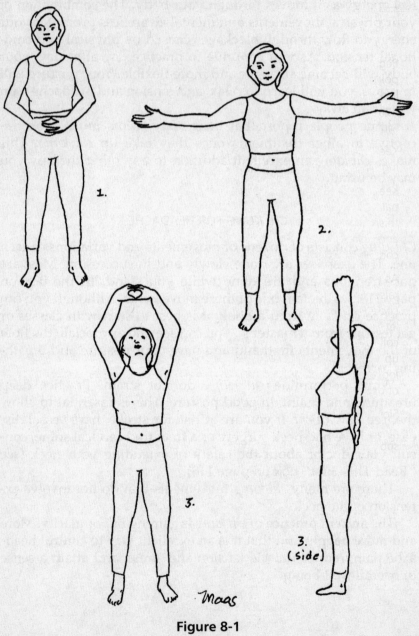

1.

2.

3.

3.
(side)

Maas

Figure 8-1

EMBRACING THE MOON

- Begin by standing with your feet at hip width under your hips, toes pointing straight ahead and knees very slightly, comfortably bent—not locked. Hold your hands over your navel, palms facing up. Keep your left hand on top of your right and let your two thumbs touch at the tips. Maintain this position for several seconds and clear your mind.

- Keep your legs and back straight, your head upright, and your eyes looking straight ahead.

- Keep your mouth closed and let your tongue curl up to a point on your palate just behind the teeth where it feels like it fits. In *chi kung* tradition, this action completes the energy circuit for the meridians in your body and acts to balance your energy. Imagine a current of energy or light coming down from the sky, through your head and tongue to your neck.

- As you inhale slowly through your nose and keep your mouth closed, raise your arms slowly out to your sides to gather the energy in a big circle around you. As you continue to lift your arms up over your head, let your middle fingertips touch each other. Imagine that your palms collect the energy of the sun. In your mind, picture your bioenergy rising up through you with your breath. If you can, lean your head back and look at your outstretched hands. Remain in this position for several seconds.

- Slowly lower your arms back to the level of your navel. As you lower your arms, release your breath slowly and release a ''ha'' that comes from a spot just below your navel. Repeat this exercise three times.

YOGA

The word *yoga* means "union," and the practice is based on the union of the self—mind, body, and spirit—with a higher consciousness. According to yogic philosophy, these three elements cannot be separated, and as humans we are linked with all things, living and inanimate.

There are many branches of yoga, and each has its own focus. The most common type in the United States is hatha yoga, which focuses on breathing exercises, sustained physical postures, increasing powers of concentration, and deep relaxation.

WHY YOGA WORKS

Yoga trains the body to remain quiet and relaxed and to create harmony within the mind and body. The overall result of practicing hatha yoga is a feeling of well-being and relaxation, flexibility, and strength. It is a tool for relaxing into and relieving the tension around pain and pain itself.

YOGA FOR HEADACHES

There are hundreds of yoga positions. We have chosen three hatha yoga exercises known to be helpful in headache relief. See Appendices I and II for where to get more information on yoga. Review the "Read This First" box on page 118 before beginning any exercises.

Before you begin, here are some general guidelines:

- Take your time: remain in each posture for at least 1 minute.
- Wear loose, comfortable clothing, and remove your shoes, belt, and constrictive jewelry.
- It is best to do yoga several hours after a meal.
- Be conscious of your breathing and keep an easy, gentle rhythm. Before you begin any kind of yoga exercise, focus on slow, diaphragmatic breathing for several minutes. This is the deep breathing technique that is the easiest to learn and is recommended by many yogic practices (refer to Chapter 7).

- Every time you exhale, feel the release of tension.
- Do only those exercises that are comfortable for you.
- Explanations of exercises are guidelines only. You may want to modify them to suit your own needs and capabilities.
- The purpose of the exercises is focused awareness, not performance. Tune in to your breathing and how your body feels.
- Use only the muscles necessary for the exercise. If other muscles tighten up, concentrate on loosening them.
- Keep your eyes closed or open, whichever is most comfortable for you. Many people prefer to close their eyes, although some find that focusing on a still or distant object is very relaxing.
- Give yourself time to end each exercise session with 5 to 10 minutes of deep relaxation (described below—The Corpse); rise slowly and gently.
- To prepare for these poses, make a comfortable place on the floor, using a blanket, towels, futon, or exercise mat.

Deep Relaxation Pose—The Corpse

The Corpse pose is a basic beginning point as well as the resting pose before and after doing other exercises. When you reach the point where you are doing many positions, use this pose to rest in between and to focus on your breathing. Do what is comfortable for you: some people use the Corpse for 3 to 5 minutes at the beginning of an exercise session, 1 to 3 minutes in between exercises, and 5 to 10 minutes at the session's end.

Lie on your back and close your eyes. Place your arms comfortably at your sides, at about a 45-degree angle to your body. Keep your fingers curled slightly and your hands relaxed with palms upward. Relax your face and breathe slowly and easily. Place your feet an easy two feet apart with your hips relaxed so your toes fall outward to the sides.

Eye Exercise

The eye exercise is especially helpful if your headache is associated with eyestrain. If you blink during any portion when the instructions ask you not to, it's okay!

- Sit on a soft, padded surface on the floor or in a chair with your feet flat on the floor. Pretend there is a large clock on the wall in front of you. Without moving your head or blinking your eyes, look up to the 12-o'clock position and then down to the 6-o'clock position. Repeat this three times, then blink several times.
- Close your eyes and relax for a moment.
- Open your eyes and look to the 3-o'clock position, then the 9-o'clock. Repeat this three times, then blink several times.
- Close your eyes and relax for a moment.
- Look at your imaginary clock again and, without blinking, look at each hour position, beginning at 12 and going clockwise. When you reach 12 again, blink several times and then close your eyes and relax.
- Open your eyes and repeat the entire sequence, this time counterclockwise. When done, close your eyes and relax.
- Rub your palms together and cup your warmed hands over your closed eyes. Feel the warmth penetrate the area around your eyes and melt the tension away.

The Plough

The Plough is a more advanced movement that stretches the entire spine. To get into the Plough, lie face up on the floor with your knees bent, feet on the ground, arms at your sides, palms down. We recommend that you place a folded towel under your shoulders to prevent neck strain, especially if you have any neck problems or past injuries. Relax for a few moments and be sure your neck is long, not crimped. If you are uncomfortable at this point, fold your arms across your chest or maintain them at your sides and practice this passive stretch until it is easy.

If you are flexible and comfortable, you can continue the exercise. Move slowly and carefully. Use your belly muscles to roll your knees toward your chest, then push up your buttocks with your hands until your knees come over the top of your head (Figure 8-2). Continue to roll as you breathe deeply and bring your knees to the sides of your head near your ears. Breathe and relax. If you can, let your knees begin to straighten. The Plough in its final form looks like drawing 3 in the illustration, with the toes on the floor. Roll back slowly to your starting position.

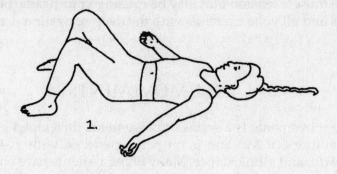

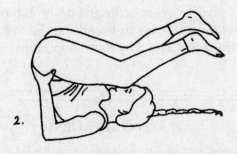

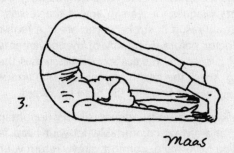

Figure 8-2

It may take years of practice to reach this full position, yet the intermediate stages of back lengthening may be all you need to undo muscle tension that may be causing your headache. Follow this and all yoga exercises with the deep relaxation (Corpse) pose.

BALANCE MOVEMENTS

Balance movements is a series of movements developed by one of the authors (P. M.) and is on her experience with yoga, *chi kung/tai chi*, and ethnic dance. Many of her patients have enjoyed headache pain relief when practicing body-in-motion. The movements are slow, easy, and enjoyable. Once you internalize them and they become automatic, you will maintain relaxation and balance during your ordinary daily activities. Begin each movement with awareness of breathing. Each movement builds on the one before it and is progressive, so it is best to do the

READ THIS FIRST

If you experience dizziness or unusual symptoms while doing any of the movements in this chapter, stop and visit your doctor for an examination. Also, some of the movements involve bending the head backward. These movements can pinch the vessels that supply blood to the brain. If there are clots, plaques, or tears in any of the vessels, bending the head backward could result in stroke. If you are in a high-risk group for stroke, see your doctor before doing any of the movements. If you are taking birth-control pills or any medication that increases the risk of vessel disease or clotting, check the health of your vertebral arteries before doing any exercise that involves bending the head backward.

To check your vertebral arteries, sit fully upright in a chair and then slowly, gently, and always comfortably, let your head fall backward so you look up. If you have any discomfort, slowly return your head to its upright position. If you have any dizziness, visual changes, or other unusual symptoms, or if you have questions about the health of your neck and blood vessels, talk to your doctor.

exercises in order as shown on the videotape (see Appendix II). However, in this chapter, we have provided explanations of several of the movements so you can experience how simple and effective they can be. They require some practice, especially those that involve awareness of muscle tension and position. Some of the movements may be completely new to you, and that is one reason they are so effective. They are designed to break up old habits you may have and shift you from a person with headache to a person without headache. Go through these movements every day to help prevent headache, or at the first sign of head pain.

WHY BALANCE MOVEMENTS WORK

Balance movements help you relieve the physical tension held in your neck and shoulders and allow you to maintain a loose, long feeling in your neck at all times. The motions involved are subtle yet powerful ways to alter body chemistry and physical structure and allow you to rebuild yourself as a person free of head pain. The videos are effective for most physical complaints. For optimal results and for complicated physical and emotional histories, seek an individualized program from a trained specialist.

BALANCE MOVEMENTS OVERVIEW

Begin each movement session by focusing on your breath. Refer to Chapter 7, where we discuss breathing techniques. If you have a favorite position for relaxation, get into that position when you practice deep breathing. Remember, if you are at risk for stroke, have vessel disease, or have had neck surgery or a fractured cervical spine, consult your doctor before beginning body-in-motion (see "Read This First" box on page 118).

When headache patients do the entire series of balance movements in the order shown on the video, many report excellent headache pain relief. The movements include those that relax the head and neck, movements for body alignment, neck stretches, and movements to improve posture. Below we have included one example movement from the many in each of these categories as a sample. These movements can be done easily at home or at work.

POSITION OF RELIEF

At the first sign of headache pain, find the position in which you feel the least discomfort. This position will be different for each person.

- Explore your options: sit, lie down, stretch, bend, or turn one way or the other.

- Breathe slowly and deeply, directing your breath to any area of stress or pain, such as the neck or shoulders.

- Experiment with staying in a darkened room, using hot or cold packs on your neck or shoulders, and/or massaging your neck and shoulders.

Sitting Forward Bend

The movement called sitting forward bend relaxes the head and neck (Figure 8-3). Sit on the edge of a chair with your feet flat on the floor, hip width apart. With your elbows resting on your knees or thighs, hang your hands between your legs. Slowly roll down your spine by nodding your head and allowing your neck and upper, middle, and lower back to curl forward. Let your arms fall between your legs and hang toward the floor. Stay in

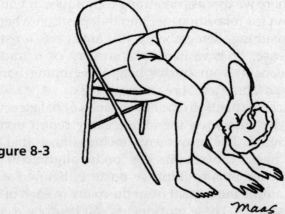

Figure 8-3

maas

that position, breathing easily, as long as you are comfortable. Then roll up by tucking your pelvis to draw your lower—then middle and upper—back upward, and then your neck and head to come into alignment. Breathe easily.

Neck Shifts

Neck shifts improve head position and loosen head and neck muscles. Do them while seated or standing, without straining, and repeat them three times. If possible, do so in front of a mirror. Without tilting your head, shift your head forward and back so that your whole face rides forward a *little* and back *a lot* with respect to your shoulders. Focus on keeping your head level with the ground. Keep your shoulders down and still. Then place your open palms on either side of your head about $1/2$ inch away from your ears. Shift your face from side to side, like a belly dancer, and touch your left ear to your left palm, then your right ear to your right palm. Repeat back and forth several times, easily, as if your neck were well lubricated. Finally, shift your head forward, to one ear, back, to the other ear, and forward, making a circle. Move slowly and smoothly, and repeat the movements in the other direction. Relax your hands on your lap. Now, imagine there is a long-handled paintbrush attached to the top of your head. Rotate your head in one direction, and then the other, as you "paint" a large circle on the ceiling.

Neck Stretches

This powerful series of neck stretches may be the single tool you need to relieve stress headaches. Read through and imagine the movements before you do them. If any movement is difficult or uncomfortable, slowly guide your head and neck away from the stretch to avoid any sudden movement to the stretched areas. Be extremely cautious and gentle throughout the movements.

If you feel any discomfort, stop and do shoulder rolls, shrug your shoulders several times, or swing your arms. Roll forward and let your neck hang free, or lie down and rest your head. *Do not* freeze: holding tight muscles rigid only increases tension. Keep muscles warm and move them as much as you can comfortably to gradually loosen any tightness. If you experience any more stress, stop the movements for another day.

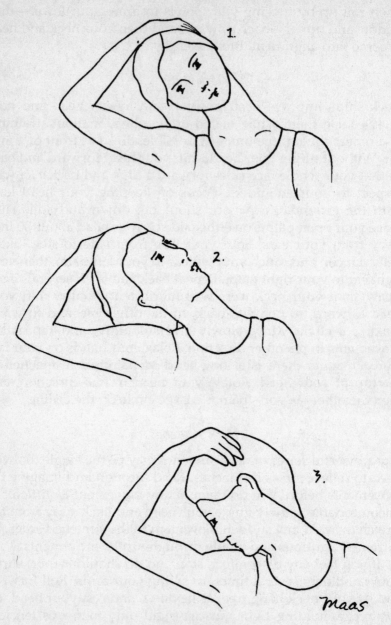

Figure 8-4

SIDE STRETCH AND ROLL

Begin with your head in a neutral position facing forward. Reach your right hand over your head and, with imaginary glue, stick it over or above your left ear. Tilt your head toward your relaxed right shoulder and let it rest there easily (Figure 8-4). Keep your head and hand in their positions and rotate your head to the right and left, pivoting on an axis that goes through the center of your head. Then let your head swing down in front of you, and roll up to the starting position. Now, switch and glue your left hand on the right side of your head, tilt your head to your relaxed left shoulder and let it rest there easily. Complete the rest of the movement as you did above.

NECK STRETCH

This is an excellent position to release tightness in the neck and to lengthen the back of the neck. Begin by kneeling on a carpeted or padded floor with your hands flat on the floor and directly below your shoulders. Bend your elbows slightly, tuck your chin, and lay the top of your head on the floor. Hold most of your weight on your hands and knees as you let your head roll back and forth, then side to side on the floor. Relax as you breathe deeply and slowly.

PUSH AND PULLEY

Begin the push-and-pulley movement with your head in a neutral, forward-facing position (Figure 8-5). Lace your fingers over the back of your head and shift your head directly back into your palms. You will feel resistance. Keep your elbows in front of you, and do not tilt your head. Feel the space between your skull and upper neck stretch a bit. "Glue" your hands to the back of your head and let your neck relax so that your head rolls forward and your elbows hang heavily down. Notice that you feel the stretch at different levels the farther down your elbows reach. Go only as far as you are comfortable at a level which needs the stretch. Now let the right elbow drop lower than the left so your head is guided by your hands to look left. Then let the left elbow drop slowly and look to the right. This is a pulley motion, which you can increase by opening your el-

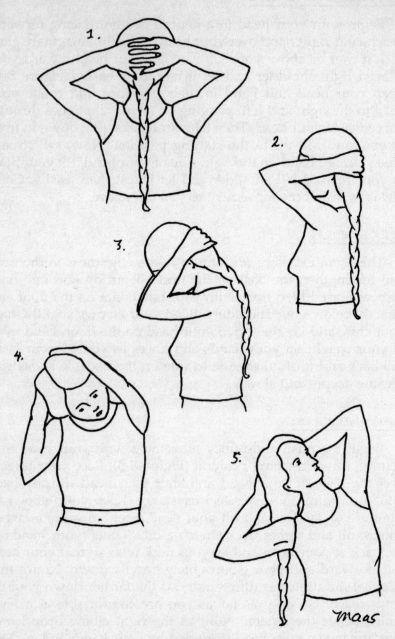

Figure 8-5

bows, one at a time, to reach up behind you. This awakens the upper back muscles, which are often frozen in people with headache.

When you are done, roll up slowly, bring your head upright and neutral, and shift your interlaced hands to the right side of your head. Hold your hands in place for resistance as you push your head into them for a few seconds. Then let your neck relax. Next, slowly lower your left ear to your left shoulder, keeping your left shoulder down and your fingers interlaced and glued to the right side of your head. Increase the stretch to your neck by first pushing gently into your hands and then stretching your neck toward your left shoulder. Repeat the push-and-stretch motion several times, then let your head roll forward and return to the neutral position. Relax your arms. Now place your interlaced fingers behind the left side of your head. Hold your hands in place for resistance and push your head into them. Repeat the motions as you did above for the right side, ultimately returning your head to the neutral position.

Balanced Stance

The balanced stance movement helps improve posture. When people think someone is checking their posture, they usually respond to old cues: chest out, chin up—the old military stance. This is not a relaxed, balanced pose. People with proper posture stand with their weight balanced on both feet, torso relaxed, with their eyes squarely attentive. Their postural "attitude" is open and centered, strong and symmetrical. Their knees are ever so slightly bent (not locked) and the pelvis is dropped. This stance also opens the channels for bioenergy to flow up the back, over the head, and down the front of the body.

The easiest way to guide someone to a balanced pose is to physically align the midpoints at each level, from the feet through the pelvis, torso, chest, shoulders, neck, and head. This concept is probably new to you, so give yourself time to feel your new centered balance. First, balance your weight between both feet, with feet apart the width of your hips. Point your toes forward as straight as is comfortable. Most people's toes point out, so keep checking on this. Let your knees bend ever so slightly, as though you are ready to go, and have a slight ease and bounce to your legs.

Most of us stand with a slightly arched lower back. This places the center of the bottom of our pelvis pointing behind us. In a natural balanced posture, the pelvis is straight and the bottom point rests directly above a spot between the feet (Figure 8-6). This pelvic move is one of the most challenging, yet also the most important, positions of alignment. Unless your pelvis is aligned, your neck and head will not find an easy neutral position. An aligned pelvis is the first step to release the back of head tension, often caused by crimping the muscles at the base of the skull, which may be causing your pain.

To align your pelvis, you may need to bend your knees a little more until this alignment is easier for you. When the pelvic girdle is upright, it feels like your guts are on a base of support within your pelvic bones instead of hanging out in front of you. Be patient; play with these images in your mind. Repetition and time are the ultimate teachers.

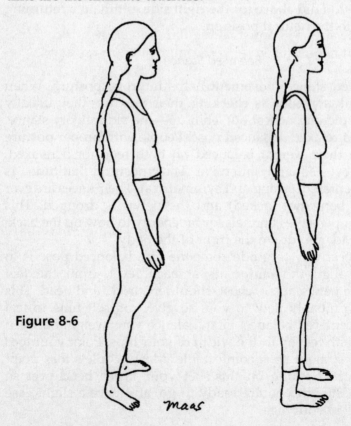

Figure 8-6

Most people have a shelf where their buttocks meet their back. See if you can rest the backs of your hands on your shelf. Gently tuck your buttocks in until the shelf disappears and your hands slide off. At first, use your stomach muscles to do the tuck. After you practice, you will release abdominal tension, feel your new center of gravity, and find your center point more easily. Once you align your pelvis, keep your feet straight, your knees flexible, and your chest, neck, head, and shoulders aligned easily on each other.

Regular practice of these balance movements can help align your body and allow all of your body fluids and your *chi* to flow more freely. Muscle tension and stress will melt away and with them, very often, your headache pain.

AEROBICS

Most people already know that regular exercise has many benefits and that aerobic exercise is recommended to prevent diabetes, depression, PMS and heart disease and to increase bone strength; even arthritis pain lessens with the right type of exercise. If you have not exercised for some time, are out of shape, or are at risk for heart disease or are diabetic, see your physician before starting any aerobic exercise program. Generally, as little as 20 minutes a day of aerobic exercise three to five days a week can help increase overall mental and physical health. The important thing is to do what you enjoy, either alone or with a friend or group: whether that be jogging, swimming, rowing, hiking, walking, biking, roller blading, cross-country skiing, or an aerobics class, you'll more likely stick with it if it's fun.

There is evidence that a very vigorous, 5- to 10-minute aerobic workout can significantly relieve cluster headache. This benefit is believed to be the result of increased serum levels of beta-endorphins, although some vascular effects also may be involved. Endorphins are chemicals present in the brain which block or alter pain perception when they are stimulated, as when you exercise. This altered perception, experienced by many athletes, is often referred to as a natural "high," a feeling of well-being.

POSTURE THERAPIES

Most of us unknowingly maintain postures that cause head-aches, back and neck pain, digestive problems, poor blood circulation, breathing disorders, arthritis, and other conditions. There are several schools of thought on how to correct these problems while living and moving with ease and good posture. We focus on two of them: the Alexander Technique and the Feldenkrais Method. The balance movement series described above has grown from these and other movement therapies that preceded it.

THE ALEXANDER TECHNIQUE

The Alexander Technique is based on the premise that our current posture is the product of years of misuse and bad habits and that we need to break those habits and learn new ones. F. Matthias Alexander, who developed his technique at the end of the nineteenth century, believed that nearly everyone has a habit of pressing his or her head back and down and compressing the spine, which can lead to a multitude of problems.

Practitioners of the Alexander Technique work with the whole body to solve specific problems with posture. Traditionally, they work one on one with individuals in lessons that last from 30 to 60 minutes. Through use of guided exercises, demonstrations of the proper way to move in everyday activities, and hands-on guidance, they help you learn to move and use your body to alleviate or eliminate pain and teach you how your body interacts with your mind. Generally, 20 to 30 lessons are needed to retrain the body and mind to work together. Wear loose, comfortable clothing during your sessions.

Although you will need to work with an Alexander Technique teacher, he or she will teach you to conduct a self-analysis for posture, which we present here. You can use these questions to evaluate your posture to determine if any of these systems of posture correction seem appropriate for you. (See Appendix I for help in finding a technique practitioner.)

To evaluate your posture, stand unclothed in front of a full-length mirror. Be as objective as possible. This is not the time to chastise yourself for eating that piece of chocolate cake. Think of yourself as a swan, graceful in motion. That is what you want to achieve. Answer the following questions about what you see in the mirror.

Front view:

- Does my head sit squarely on my shoulders?
- Do I cock my head to one side?
- Does my chin jut too far forward?
- Does my neck extend out in front of my body?
- Am I shrugging my shoulders?
- Do I have one shoulder higher than the other?
- Are my shoulders rounded forward?
- Do I draw in my chest?
- Do I stand rigidly with my chest up high?
- Is one hip higher than the other?
- Do my arms hang evenly?

Side view:

- Do I overarch my back?
- Do I hold my buttocks in too tight?
- Does my stomach form a little shelf?
- Do I try to suck in my stomach?

Misalignments can cause and affect the patterns of stress and tension you carry with you. Alexander Technique teachers help you become aware of the movements and postures you need to change and then show you how: how to sit, drive, talk on the phone, stand, lift, and lie down correctly. They can help you rearrange your workplace to minimize stress. Kathleen Ballard, chairperson of the Society of Teachers of the Alexander Technique, sums up the lessons this way: "By words and subtle, informed touch, pupils are taught how to allow the neck to be free, the head to be released forward and up, and the back to lengthen and widen. They learn how to promote this lengthening and freedom when moving from standing to sitting and vice versa. The teacher's touch and advice help the pupils become aware of habitual misuse and enables them to make changes."

FELDENKRAIS METHOD

The Feldenkrais Method had its beginnings in the Alexander Technique, when Moshe Feldenkrais, an engineer by trade, became interested in holistic health and the human body in motion. Feldenkrais believed that people learn just enough physical movement to function and leave much of their potential undeveloped. Like practitioners of the Alexander Technique, those trained in the Feldenkrais Method emphasize that their role is to teach you to move your body in ways that will become like second nature to you and to help you reach your physical potential. This approach has been very successful in treating chronic headache pain, relieving muscle tension, improving posture, and increasing flexibility.

The Feldenkrais Method consists of more than 1,000 different exercises or movements. Many of the exercises are done on a padded table or on the floor, where your teacher will guide you into movements that are easy, slow, and without strain or pain. To allow maximum movement, wear loose, comfortable clothing for your lessons. Each movement is designed to increase your awareness of your body and the communication between it and your mind. Lessons typically last 30 to 50 minutes, and you may need 12 to 24 lessons over a 4- to 12-week period, depending on your physical state when you begin.

Movement therapy is an excellent way to relieve muscle tension, increase body awareness, improve posture, promote blood circulation, and increase flexibility—all of which work to relieve headache pain. You may want to practice one or more techniques in this chapter and combine them with other natural approaches given in this book. You will likely discover that whatever movement therapy you choose, you will not only enjoy headache pain relief, but you also will experience an overall feeling of well-being and balance.

9

ACUPUNCTURE AND OTHER BIOENERGY THERAPIES

Some people call it the "life force"; others refer to it as "vitality." In Ayurvedic, it is *prana*; in yogic, *kundalini*; in Japanese, *ki*; in Taoist, *chi* (pronounced "chee" or "key"). All of these terms can be used interchangeably to refer to bioenergy.

Bioenergy is an invisible but vital force that flows through all human beings. It is intimately associated with the flow of blood, lymph, and normalization of all body functions; balancing the flow brings about headache pain relief. The balance of energy maintains our physical, emotional, mental, and spiritual functioning. To do this effectively, it must move freely along certain paths, or *meridians*, throughout the body. Each meridian passes through many parts of the body and has many points, like "connect the dots," which identify the energy paths. These points are where practitioners of various bioenergy therapies—which include acupuncture, acupressure (shiatsu), Oriental massage, polarity therapy, reflexology, and therapeutic touch—use touch or other means to open blockages and balance bioenergy so it can travel unhindered along the meridians and maintain a person in a state of well-being and health. This chapter explains the techniques used to balance energy flow for each of these therapies and explores how these therapies can be used to treat and prevent headache.

ACUPRESSURE/*SHIATSU*

Acupressure is the application of finger pressure to specific points on the body in order to influence the flow of bioenergy. These points are sometimes referred to as "kernels" of tension that lie within tight muscles. There are several names and variations for treatments that are similar to acupressure, including *shiatsu, Do-In,* and *G-Jo.* These and other pressure-point therapies have a similar approach and often similar points for treatment, yet there are some differences. Some acupressure therapists, for example, also may use their palms, elbows, knees, and feet to affect pressure on the points. Acupressure therapists and *shiatsu* practitioners vary in how hard and how long they press the points and the type of movements they use. Acupressure can provide significant relief of migraine, sinus headache, and temporomandibular joint (TMJ) syndrome, and it often eliminates the pain of tension headache or headache that accompanies colds or flu.

HOW DOES ACUPRESSURE WORK?

As your bioenergy moves through the meridians in your body, sometimes it becomes blocked, often due to stress or muscle tension. Acupressure, like acupuncture, releases that blocked bioenergy flow and helps return your body to a balanced state.

TREATING YOURSELF USING PRESSURE POINTS

In most cases, it is completely safe to self-treat with acupressure. For a few medical conditions, however, acupressure should be avoided. As a precaution, do not push hard or directly on injured or fragile tissues, including skin sores, fractured or weak bones, infections, or vessels that are clotted, especially if you have a history or risk of blood clots or hemorrhage. In pregnancy, avoid pressure points on the leg and the perineum (between the anus and vagina), which acupressure therapists say can increase the chance of miscarriage.

You can easily learn pressure-point techniques to help your own pain and that of your friends and family. There are many good books and classes, but the best way to start is with a trained practitioner, who will treat you to a new, enjoyable, possibly curative experience.

Feel free to try a few of the points illustrated in Figure 9-1. Use the tip of your strongest finger—probably your thumb—and find the point or "kernel" of tension within any muscle that feels tight. Press into the center of the kernel hard enough so that it "hurts good" and you can relax around the sensation before you slowly release. Breathe easily and remain calm throughout. Press on each point for two to three minutes. You can enlist the help of a friend for points you can't reach.

The relief points illustrated can be used for all types of headache. One key acupressure point (A) found in the web space between your index finger and thumb close to the hand bone leading to the index finger is commonly recommended to relieve headache accompanied by constipation. Also apply pressure to points around the eye socket (B), especially on the affected side. The points on and to the side of the nose may be helpful in relieving sinusitis (B). Press into the tender points underneath the base of your skull on either side of the spinal column (D). There are many techniques to apply pressure here—with your thumbs or fingertips; by lying down on two rubber balls tied in a sock; or by using the rounded upper edge of a chair back. Or a friend can gently cradle your head while applying pressure with his or her fingertips.

You or your friend can also find and press any tight, tender points on your head, scalp, forehead, and along the back of your neck.

YOUR VISIT TO AN ACUPRESSURE THERAPIST

On your first visit, wear comfortable, loose-fitting clothing. The practitioner will ask you about your medical and personal history and check your pulse. The acupressure will probably be done while you lie on a padded massage or treatment table or on a futon. During the session, which generally lasts about one hour, you may be asked to lie on your stomach, your side, and your back. One or more sessions with an acupressure therapist will allow you to become familiar with the points to press when you treat yourself.

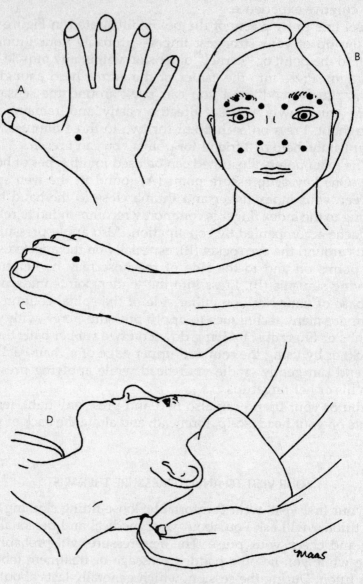

Figure 9-1

ACUPUNCTURE

Acupuncture, from the Latin *acus* (needle) and *punctura* (to prick) is an ancient healing and pain-management therapy that has been traced back to the sixth century B.C. in China. Acupuncturists use sharp, skinny needles to puncture the skin at precisely defined points along the meridians, or energy pathways in the body, in order to open up the flow of bioenergy, relieve pain, and restore good health and harmony.

HOW DOES ACUPUNCTURE WORK?

When an acupuncture needle is inserted into a specific point, it opens up areas in the body where energy is blocked. Western science lacks adequate ways to measure or explain these effects, and thus some people say acupuncture works because of the placebo effect—basically, because people *believe* it will work. However, acupuncture relieves pain in skeptics, children, and animals and has many other profound health benefits.

Several theories have been suggested. One theory is that the needles send so many intense but nonpainful messages to the spinal cord and brain that the pain messages cannot get through. Another idea is that the needles stimulate the production and release of endorphins and enkephalins, the body's own pain-suppressing chemicals. This theory is supported by the finding of an increased level of endorphins in the cerebrospinal fluid after acupuncture treatment. Many people feel euphoric for hours, and some for weeks, after an acupuncture treatment. For people with chronic pain, sometimes the greatest relief comes one or two days after the treatment.

ACUPUNCTURE FOR HEADACHES AND MIGRAINES

You will need to go to a professional acupuncturist for treatments. See Appendix I for information on how to locate a practitioner in your area.

Acupuncturists use several different methods to determine where the energy is blocked. In addition to questions about medical history and symptoms, they observe eyes, skin, face, tongue, and overall general appearance. The Chinese maintain that the color, texture, and shape of the tongue, for example, can reveal where problems may lie. Questions about eating habits and any elimination problems are common, and they listen to the voice, breathing, and coughing and note any breath odor. They also use pulse diagnosis, a method that allows them to determine the state of the body's energy in the meridians by feeling the radial artery pulse in the wrist. Trained acupuncturists typically check nine different pulses on each wrist and identify which areas of the body have a disturbance. They can tell, for example, if a migraine may be caused in part by a problem in the stomach or large intestine by reading the pulse for that meridian.

An instrument called a *ryodoraku* can provide similar information. While you hold onto a small metal cylinder, the acupuncturist uses a pencil-like tool attached to a monitoring device to measure the resistance of specific points along the meridians by touching the point of the *ryodoraku* to the skin and checking the reading on the monitor. Other symptoms and findings suggest problems along meridians or organ system lines.

The needles used in acupuncture are commonly made of stainless steel or a silver alloy and vary in length. After the needles are inserted to various depths through the skin, some practitioners rotate the needles between their fingers, quickly or slowly in one direction or another, while others simply insert and remove them, depending on whether the area needs stimulation and if so, what type. Another popular technique is to connect an electric stimulator to the needles to deliver a low-voltage current. Some practitioners say this electroacupuncture technique greatly improves the effectiveness of the treatment.

Some people feel little or no pain; others are uncomfortable at some times and at some points. Many people feel a pulse of energy flow or release of tension. Needles usually are left in place for 20 minutes or longer. After treatment, individuals usually feel balanced and refreshed—a feeling that can last hours to weeks.

To treat headaches, needles are commonly placed in the middle of the web area on the hands between the thumb and index finger (referred to as Li-4), points on either side of the nose

(St-3), a point at the base of the skull (GB-20), and a point between the large toe and the one next to it (Liv-3) (see Figure 9-1). Needle placement in these points has brought people relief from tension headaches, migraines, and headaches associated with TMJ syndrome and trigeminal neuralgia (see Chapter 5). Results of several controlled studies show that overall, acupuncture treatments are effective in approximately 75 percent of cases.

Depending on the type and severity of headache, you may feel relief immediately or within a few hours of an acupuncture treatment. Some people need to return for six to eight treatments before they get lasting improvement, although others have no pain after two or three treatments. The treatment plan is as unique as you and your headache are. Acupuncture is very effective for acute and recurrent sinusitis and the headache pain that accompanies it, typically providing results immediately or within hours that last the entire season. A series of treatments may offer an even longer effect.

ORIENTAL MASSAGE

Unlike some Western massage techniques such as Swedish massage (discussed in Chapter 10), which is based on physical, biological principles, Oriental massage is based primarily on the premise that massage moves and balances bioenergy, or *chi*, in the Chinese tradition. Oriental massage promotes the free flow of bioenergy in the body by opening up areas where it has become congested. Oriental massage does not involve oils and can be done through clothing.

Oriental massage is effective in the treatment of tension headaches, migraines, and headaches associated with the common cold, flu, neuralgia, arthritis, and other medical conditions. There are two basic approaches to Oriental massage. In *amma*, gentle strokes and mild pressure are used, which relieve simple stress and tension. In *tui na*, practitioners gently but vigorously rub, tap, press, push, squeeze, twist, and roll to move *chi* and treat problems such as stiff joints. *Tui na* also includes joint mobilization, which is sometimes similar to osteopathic manipulation.

HOW DOES ORIENTAL MASSAGE WORK?

Both *amma* and *tui na* awaken the energy at pressure points and stimulate movement of the *chi*. Unlike Swedish massage, in which the therapists focus the direction of their massage so blood flow toward the heart is increased, practitioners of Oriental massage make their moves away from the heart to release blocked energy. As the therapist works the points along the meridian lines, he or she focuses on each point and concentrates on connecting his consciousness and his energy with yours. To practitioners of Oriental bodywork, this connection is essential for healing to occur. (See Appendix I for information on how to find a certified Oriental massage practitioner.)

ORIENTAL MASSAGE FOR HEADACHES: SELF-TREATMENT

Oriental massage therapists often incorporate many types of massage techniques during a session. Following is a simplified version that you can do for yourself for your headache pain. Apply only the amount of pressure that is comfortable. Refer to Figure 9-2 for point positions.

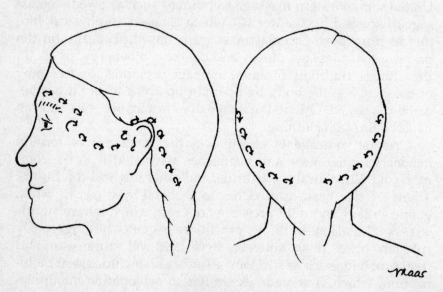

Figure 9-2

Choose a quiet place where you won't be disturbed for about 15 minutes and sit in a comfortable chair.

- Using the thumb, index, and middle fingers of both your hands, *gently* knead your eyeball in a circular motion, about eight times in each direction. (Skip this step if you wear hard contact lenses, have glaucoma or other eye problems, or have a very slow pulse or low blood pressure.

- Take the middle fingers of both hands and make little circles in both directions just to the side of your eyes. Make circles away from the eyes and then toward the eyes.

- With the tips of both middle fingers, make a series of dragging motions, like little nudges beginning from above and between your eyebrows outward to the points just to the sides of your eyes. Continue along the cheekbones on both sides of your head and around your ears to the points at your back hairline that lie about 1 to 2 inches on either side of your spine. Do this six times, three times with each hand.

- Make your nudges and circles firm but gentle and push mostly outward and downward, as though drawing tension from the front to the back. When you get there, spend extra time massaging the base of the skull. Repeat many times, as long as you feel as if the massage is relieving tension.

- You can also work the points around your skull with a "press and lift" technique. Place one palm with your fingers pointing up on the center of your forehead and the other palm at the base of your skull in the back of your head. Using soft, flat palms, squeeze in firmly for one second, then lift your palms, move them each $1/4$ to $1/2$ inch around your head in the same direction. When the front palm gets to the back and the back palm gets to the front, repeat in the other direction without breaking an easy, gentle rhythm. Repeat as many times as feels good.

PROFESSIONAL ORIENTAL MASSAGE

As with other forms of holistic therapy, professional Oriental massage therapists work to balance the entire body, as head pain is seen as a symptom of imbalance. Therefore, regardless of the type of headache you have, you will receive a treatment for overall tension.

POLARITY THERAPY

The head has a positive charge, the feet a negative charge, and the life force constantly flows through these two points along five specific pathways. This is what Dr. Randolph Stone, an osteopath, chiropractor, naturopath, and founder of polarity therapy, believed, as do those who practice this therapy today. Polarity therapy is based on the idea that pain is a manifestation of blocked electromagnetic energy. Dr. Stone described five energy centers in the body that he said must be in balance in order for the life force to flow unhindered (Figure 9-3).

A polarity therapy program involves three basic concepts—bodywork (manipulation), stretching exercises, and diet—all of which work together to eliminate or reduce pain and restore the energy flow. Polarity therapy incorporates what Dr. Stone believed to be the best from the many therapeutic techniques he studied: reflexology, craniosacral therapy, deep massage, and Ayurvedic medicine (a system of philosophy and medicine from India).

HOW DOES POLARITY THERAPY WORK?

Like other energy therapies, polarity therapy works by moving bioenergy through areas where it is blocked. Polarity bodywork alone will probably relieve your headache pain; however, polarity therapists also consult on the other two concepts of polarity therapy—exercise and diet—as the combination of all three factors is more likely to bring you complete and lasting relief.

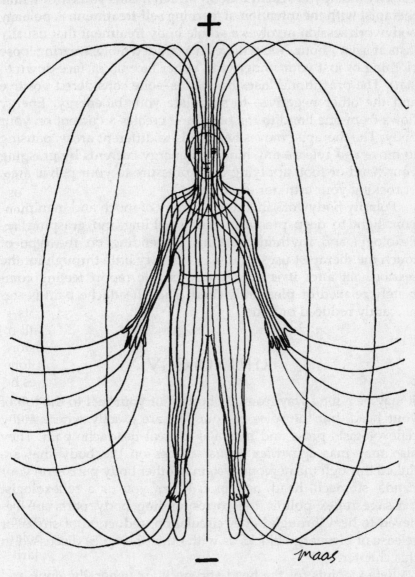

Figure 9-3

POLARITY THERAPY FOR HEADACHE

Polarity therapy is "client based," which means you work with a therapist with the intention of learning self-treatment. A polarity bodywork session involves a whole-body treatment that usually lasts at least 1 hour. You will lie on a padded table, wearing loose clothing or just your underwear, either face up or face down to start. The practitioner uses her hands—one considered positive and the other negative—to stimulate your bioenergy. Energy flows from one hand to the other and creates a current on your body. The therapist moves her hands to different areas, pausing to move and release any hindered energy currents by grasping your hand or foot, applying deep pressure to your pelvic area, or rocking your arm, for example.

Polarity bodywork involves a variety of touch and manipulation: light to deep pressure, gentle holding and grasping, reflexology, and rhythmic rocking. Depending on the type of touch the therapist uses, you may feel very little throughout the session. Yet after it is over, many people report feeling completely relaxed or pleasantly tired. Their headache pain is significantly reduced or gone.

REFLEXOLOGY

It may be a long way from the bottom of your feet to the top of your head, but the soles of your feet are exactly where many reflexologists press and massage to treat headache pain. They also may massage *reflex points*—places on the body that are linked through the nervous system to other body parts—on your hands, stomach, head, and face. When you or a reflexologist massage reflex points, the corresponding body parts are believed to heal through better circulation, reduction of stress, or release of bioenergy blocks as with other therapies discussed in this chapter.

Reflex points for the head and neck are generally along and between the toes. Beyond that, not all systems involving referral points for distant organs and body regions are consistent. One will indicate sinus points in the web spaces of hands and feet, and another source will show them on the tips of the toes (see Figure 9-4). Use the tips of your fingers or knuckles, even your

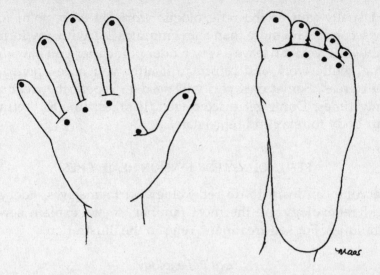

Figure 9-4

elbows (sitting tailor fashion) to explore the bottoms and tops of both feet. Your headache may be due to constipation, back strain, or another area that may have a corresponding sore reflex point on your feet or hands. Finding the sore reflex can help with your diagnosis! If you would like more detailed information, reflexology charts are available through the International Institute of Reflexology (see Appendix I).

HOW DOES REFLEXOLOGY WORK?

Reflexology is a type of pressure-point massage that focuses on tender or painful energy points throughout the body that correspond to other distant sites and organs. Theoretically, reflexology is similar to Oriental meridian therapies such as acupressure and acupuncture. All of these systems are based on the belief that they are effective because they cause endorphin release, increase bioenergy flow, stimulate the flow of blood and lymph, and follow the idea that any part of the body completely reflects the whole. Many people find that foot and hand massage can be as relaxing and beneficial as an entire body massage. When you work all the reflex points on one part of the body, such as your feet, you open up all the reflex points in your body and flood your entire body with healing energy.

Usually you or the reflexologist work on each point for a few seconds—no more than a few minutes. As with any form of bodywork, you can leave a very tender point after you have done some gentle work and return to it after you have opened up other areas. Sometimes you will need to repeat the treatment many times. Don't get discouraged. It takes time to "retrain" your body to relax and rejuvenate.

REFLEXOLOGY FOR TENSION HEADACHES

Everyone can learn to do reflexology on themselves. Foot and hand reflexology are the most familiar, so we explain several techniques. For self-treatment, refer to the illustration.

Foot Reflexology

You can perform foot reflexology as follows:

- Find a comfortable, quiet place where you can sit undisturbed for about 15 minutes.
- Reflexology is usually done without lubrication, however some therapists suggest using a greaseless lotion or powder on the feet.
- Grasp the heel, toes, or ankle of your left foot with your left hand and place the thumb of your right hand on the sole of your foot at the heel. As you keep your thumb slightly bent at the joint, apply steady, even pressure with your thumb as you move it along in a forward, kneading motion, beginning at your heel (see Figure 9-4) and moving toward your toes: press one spot, release; move slightly toward the toes, press again; and so on. When you reach the ball of your foot, return to the heel and start from a new spot. Once you have covered the entire bottom of your sole, massage the base pads and tips of all your toes and between the toes. Tuck your fingertips between the web spaces of your toes. This may help relieve sinus pain. Use your fingers to apply the same pressure on the top of your foot.
- Repeat the entire sequence as often as you like.
- Focus on any tender spots.

Hand Reflexology

As with the foot, there are points on the hand that, when rubbed, can relieve head pain. Beginning at the pad of your thumb, massage firmly. Squeeze the sides of your thumb on either side of the nail and massage just below the thumbnail on the top of the thumb. Keep searching for tender spots; when you find one, massage it for seconds to minutes.

Use your thumb and forefinger of one hand to pinch and massage the web area (Figure 9-4) between your thumb and forefinger of the other hand. Massage the entire area up to where the bones come together. If you find any tender spots, rub them slowly and gently. Breathe deeply—they can be very tender. There are also powerful trigger points to release neck pain at the webs between the fourth and fifth fingers of either hand (Figure 9-4). Press these spots between your thumb and index finger, and massage them gently for several minutes. Many people prefer reflexology over other touch therapies because it doesn't require them to get undressed or to have someone touching them except for their hands or feet. Reflexology is easy to do for yourself and, once you know the points, you can do it anywhere—while watching television or at your desk during a break at work.

THERAPEUTIC TOUCH

We have already talked about the energy that flows *within* you. Therapeutic touch deals with the energy that extends *beyond* your body like an energy field. Although this concept may sound bizarre, therapeutic touch has proved efficacy and is taught in leading medical and nursing schools across the United States. Nurses use this technique every day in hospitals around the world.

Therapeutic touch became popular in the United States thanks to a registered nurse named Dolores Krieger, Ph.D., a professor of nursing at New York University who introduced this therapy in 1975. Since then, it's been shown to reduce headache pain by up to 70 percent. It is particularly successful in reducing headache pain associated with stress, menstruation, and fatigue.

HOW DOES THERAPEUTIC TOUCH WORK?

Many people who experience the power of therapeutic touch say it leaves them remarkably relaxed and feeling much less or no pain. But how does it do that? Therapeutic touch practitioners believe life energy flows from their hands into the energy field of their patients. The patients internalize the energy and allow it to balance their own disturbed, weak, or congested energy field. Once the energy is in balance, the body can heal itself.

If you don't feel better the first time you try therapeutic touch, try again! Connecting with your energy may take some time.

THERAPEUTIC TOUCH FOR YOUR HEADACHE

You and a friend may want to take a class in therapeutic touch so you can help each other. There are excellent books on the subject, including the classic written by Dr. Krieger herself (see Sources and Suggested Readings). However, to best learn therapeutic touch, you need to receive instruction from a professional therapist, who can explain the sensations you will feel as you learn this technique.

The following is an overview of the basic steps involved in therapeutic touch, which will give you a general idea of what occurs during a session. The therapist conducts the entire session by moving her or his hands in the energy field that surrounds your body; thus, there is no direct skin contact in therapeutic touch.

1. *Centering:* The first step is centering: those who perform therapeutic touch must clear their mind and focus on their personal energy source. To do this, they may close their eyes, breathe deeply, and picture themselves as energy or as receiving energy from above or another source, or they may use whatever technique works for them. Once they are at peace, they are ready to assess your energy field.
2. *Assessment:* The assessment can be done in whatever position is most practical and comfortable for both you and the therapist. She will hold her hands, palms toward you, 1 to 3 inches away from your body. With one hand in front of you and the other in back of you, or with both hands in

front or in back, she will pass her hands down your body from head to toe. The therapist notes subtle changes in temperature or any vibration that indicates a congested or weakened area of energy flow, such as a backache, an infection, or a healed wound.

3. *Clearing congestion:* To break up any blocked energy, the therapist will make repeated sweeping motions down-ward with her hands and move the energy away from your body after each sweep. This is done for your entire body.

4. *Balancing the energy field:* As energy is unblocked and moved, your energy field regains its normal flow, because your body inherently wants to be balanced and whole. The therapist will pass her hands over your entire energy field one final time to ensure that balance has been achieved.

To use therapeutic touch on yourself, first center yourself. Imagine energy is flowing into your body and empowering you. Then place your hands over the area you want to heal and visu-alize the energy flowing out of your hands into that area. Main-tain this visualization for at least 3 to 5 minutes, or until the pain is reduced or disappears.

Whether you have someone else do therapeutic touch for you or you do it yourself, allow yourself to remain open to the expe-rience. It may take more than one session for you to get pain relief.

This chapter has presented techniques to regain and main-tain your bioenergy flow, which helps to prevent and treat head-ache pain. Even if you are somewhat skeptical about any of these therapies, we suggest you consider them—thousands of people use them every day—and enjoy natural headache pain relief.

10

OSTEOPATHY AND OTHER PHYSICAL REMEDIES

Touch and manipulative therapies have been an important part of healing since ancient times. Headache pain responds to both approaches. In this chapter, we look at how chiropractic, craniosacral therapy, hydrotherapy, myotherapy, osteopathy, physical therapy, Swedish massage, and transcutaneous electrical nerve stimulation (TENS) are used to prevent and treat head pain.

From the moment we are born, our bodies take years of physical and emotional abuse. Incidents big and small—wearing tight shoes, breaking an ankle, clenching our fists, falling off a bicycle, cradling a telephone receiver between our ear and shoulder—affect the posture, movement, and holding patterns that define our structure, behavior, and perception. The therapies presented in this chapter are similar in that each one in its own unique way works to release muscle tension and rigidity, which are the cause of most headache pain.

CHIROPRACTIC

"In case of illness, look to the spine first." The words of Hippocrates seem to be custom made for the practice of chiropractic. Chiropractic is based on the theory that much, if not most, pain is caused by dislocations of the vertebrae and joints and that normal functioning of the nervous system is essential for good health. Within the discipline, some chiropractors also incorporate nutritional concepts into their treatment programs.

Chiropractors work primarily on the musculoskeletal causes of disease. Chiropractic adjustment returns the vertebrae and joints to a normal or more functional condition so the body can heal itself. Chiropractors are not licensed physicians, however; therefore, their education and scope of practice are more limited than those of osteopaths. (See Osteopathy, page 157.)

HOW DOES CHIROPRACTIC WORK?

Chiropractic treatments are based on spinal anatomy and the fact that different parts of the spine send nerve fibers to specific parts of the body. Interference with nerve signals affects the physiology in the areas served by the affected nerves. To reduce or eliminate a pain in your head, chiropractors manipulate the area of the spine that corresponds to the location of the pain, realigning the vertebrae and relieving pressure or tension on the nerves and spinal column. You may need a series of treatments, depending on the severity and cause of your headache.

CHIROPRACTIC AND HEADACHE PAIN

Chiropractic is not a self-treatment; see How to Choose a Chiropractor in Appendix I for help in locating a chiropractor. Chiropractic has had much success in the treatment of people with tension headaches, migraines, or headaches due to poor posture or whiplash. The initial evaluation visit to a chiropractor typically includes giving a medical history and undergoing a physical examination. The chiropractor usually feels along the spine, searching for any tender spots. To rule out physical problems, chiropractors frequently take a spinal x-ray and sometimes a complete body x-ray from head to toe.

Chiropractic treatments are typically called *adjustments* and usually are done with the palms or mechanical devices. Some chiropractors use gentle manipulation while others utilize sudden, thrusting maneuvers to move bones back into place. You may be treated with a combination of both methods.

CRANIOSACRAL THERAPY

Craniosacral therapy is a type of osteopathic manipulation in which a trained therapist relieves pressure and tension in the head by making subtle adjustments to the skull, sacrum (broad spinal area above the tail bone), or other parts of the body. By feeling with their hands and watching subtle body movements, craniosacral therapists "read" the flow of cerebrospinal fluid and other fluids in the body. When they find areas where the flow is blocked, they make very gentle corrections to release the flow. Tension headaches, migraines, and cluster headaches respond well to this therapy.

HOW DOES CRANIOSACRAL THERAPY WORK?

While most conventional physicians believe the bones in the skull are immobile, proponents of craniosacral therapy say that, with training, one can detect subtle yet measurable craniosacral movement. The movement is said to be in synch with the body's pumping of cerebrospinal fluid deep within the ventricles of the brain. This flow of fluid surrounds the nervous system in a circulation separate from the body's other circulatory systems.

Craniosacral practitioners believe that any trauma to the head, beginning with the trip down the birth canal, can cause misalignment of the bones in the skull. These bones are held together by connective tissue along suture lines that allow flexibility of the skull into adulthood. It is along the suture lines that craniosacral therapists realign and remove stresses that have accumulated in the supporting membranes of the brain.

CRANIOSACRAL THERAPY FOR HEADACHE

Craniosacral therapy is not a do-it-yourself therapy; it's very specialized and results depend on the training and experience of the practitioner. Osteopaths who specialize in craniosacral therapy undergo meticulous training in the anatomy and biomechanics of cranial bone movement in addition to their medical training as physicians. Most are members of the Cranial Academy, and some have board certification. Craniosacral therapy is a true healing art and it is worthwhile to find a proficient practitioner, who may or may not also be an osteopath. See Appendix I for information on how to find an appropriate practitioner.

A typical session with a craniosacral therapist may involve the following. After you lie on your back on the treatment table, the therapist will gently and very lightly grasp your head from behind. The bones of the skull move in a contraction-expansion rhythm. When the bones are not moving in synch, the practitioner usually can feel something pulling awry. He or she can either "ride" this pull to its extreme, hold it there, and follow it as it returns to a normal rhythm, or directly guide the imbalanced motion back to normal using a very subtle, yet very powerful pull with the hands.

In many individuals, this simple head-hold manipulation causes their breathing to deepen almost immediately. Their voices are lower, their movements calmer, and they feel much more balanced and relaxed. People with chronic headache usually require a series of treatments based on the kind of pain they are experiencing. The type of holds and gentle guidance to the bones are highly individual. In most cases, headache relief occurs at the first treatment; however, additional visits and certain exercises are usually needed for long-term relief.

HYDROTHERAPY

The healing power of water, when taken internally or when experienced externally as cold water or ice or hot water or steam, has been reported since before Hippocrates. Bathing in mineral water, thermal springs, or salt-water baths or using the steam of a sauna has been credited with healing a multitude of ailments such as headache, arthritis, back pain, rheumatism, indigestion, and respiratory troubles, for many reasons.

HOW DOES HYDROTHERAPY WORK?

As your environment changes, a thermostat in your brain maintains a balance between heat gain and heat loss. If you submerge yourself in a tub of hot water, your blood vessels dilate and your pulse rate increases to maintain flow. Even though the heart works a little harder, adrenaline and thyroid hormone secretions are inhibited and you feel relaxed.

When cold water is the stimulus, your body tries to prevent heat loss by constricting your blood vessels. To produce more heat, your muscles may contract automatically in a shiver. The secretion of adrenaline and thyroid hormones increases and your heart rate and blood pressure go up.

Thus, switching back and forth between hot and cold water makes your blood vessels dilate and then constrict, and this pumping action stimulates blood circulation. Hot water applied to the feet or hands causes blood to flow to the distant dilated vessels and decreases the amount of pressure in the blood vessels elsewhere, including the brain. As the pressure decreases, pressure pain is relieved.

HYDROTHERAPY FOR HEADACHE PAIN

The following hydrotherapy treatments are for tension headaches as well as for migraine headache types accompanied by fever or nausea. These techniques, which significantly change body temperature, are old naturopathic methods for fever and are safe unless you use water that is hotter than 103 degrees Fahrenheit. If you have a heart condition or high blood pressure, suffer from seizures, are at risk for stroke, or have other medical concerns, talk with your doctor before trying these treatments.

Hot-Cold Treatment

You need a combination bathtub-shower for this treatment. Fill the tub with enough hot water to cover you when you sit and lean back, and add Epsom salts according to directions on the box. Swish the salts to dissolve them and then soak in the tub for as long as you like. Spend this time relaxing, meditating, or doing deep breathing. Play soothing music, or at least shut out distracting noise. Let your tension and worries melt into the water. When you are ready, let the water drain out, carefully step out of the tub, and dry off gently. Stay warm and relaxed; wrap yourself in a towel or robe to avoid getting chilled. After about 10 minutes (use this time to prepare hot and cold packs for later), step back into the tub for a cold, full-pressure shower. Let the water hit your feet, legs, back, front, and then your head.

After a few minutes, turn off the water, dry off quickly, and dress in warm bedclothes. Lie in bed with an ice pack on your head and a hot-water bottle at your feet for 20 minutes. After you remove the cold and hot applications, relax and sleep.

Variation for Migraines

A variation of this approach, used to alleviate migraine pain, is to alternate hot and cold showers, each lasting about three to five minutes. It is believed the temperature contrast interrupts the constriction and dilation of the blood vessels that is associated with migraines.

Head-to-Toes Treatment

Here is a remedy so simple you may be tempted to say it couldn't possibly work—but many people say it brings relief, especially for sinus-type headaches. Get a bucket or small tub that your feet can fit into comfortably. Pour in enough hot water (as hot as you can tolerate) to cover your feet. Sit with your feet in the tub and place an ice pack on your forehead and another on the back of your neck. If possible, lean back in a comfortable chair and relax deeply. Have a friend add more hot water after about 15 or 20 minutes as the water cools down. According to Peter de Vries, a hydrotherapist with the Weimar Institute, this method works because it attracts "congestion toward the feet, and away from the head."

Hydrotherapy is a good example of how therapy does not need to be complicated or expensive in order to be effective. Using the power of one of our most basic elements—water—you can enjoy headache relief.

MYOTHERAPY

Myotherapy (also called trigger-point myotherapy) is a hands-on treatment based on the concept that applying pressure to *trigger points*—injured or irritated spots in the muscles—can significantly reduce or eliminate pain. Trigger points are caused by a fall, strain, sprain, bump—any number or variety of incidents you may or may not remember or be aware of.

WHY DOES MYOTHERAPY WORK?

Myotherapists believe that the trigger points do not cause any problems until an event such as stress, an automobile accident, overexertion, or simply sleeping in an awkward position irritates them. The result is pain—if not at the trigger point location, then at another area of the body, which is where the trigger point "refers" the pain.

Bonnie Prudden, director of the Institute for Physical Fitness and Myotherapy in Tucson, Arizona, once asked myotherapy pioneer Dr. Janet Travell why myotherapy works; she replied, "You are denying the trigger point oxygen." Deep pressure on trigger points can restore the blood flow, which carries oxygen to the starving muscle.

WHAT SHOULD I EXPECT FROM A MYOTHERAPIST?

The term *myotherapy* is generic and can be used by anyone who has learned the technique. There are two types of myotherapists: those who have been trained at a certified myotherapy school and those who received their training from other sources. *Certified* myotherapists will treat only individuals who have been referred to them by a physician. Lack of certification does not necessarily mean a myotherapist is less experienced or qualified; however, certification does guarantee a standard of education (see Appendix I for information on myotherapists).

A session typically lasts 90 minutes and involves a series of deep elbow or hand pressure on tender muscles. For several days afterward, you will probably feel a slight soreness and a feeling like your muscles want to return to their old tense position. Stretching and exercise are usually recommended after treatments in order to keep the muscles limber. Each subsequent treatment will further train your muscles to remain in their proper position. Some people get headache relief after one or two treatments; others return periodically for "boosters."

MYOTHERAPY AND HEADACHE

According to myotherapists, five different regions of the head and face can be treated if you suffer from headaches, including trigger points in more than 15 muscles around the eyes and in the face, neck, and shoulders. Headache can come from distant and smaller muscles. However, the vast majority of tension headaches come from the major muscles shown in the illustration. You or a friend can massage these muscles to release tension, which usually brings at least some and often complete relief, no matter what type of headache you are suffering from. Hunt for tight, tender spots within the muscle and rub them in little circles or hold them with varying amounts of fingertip pressure. For some people, a light touch is all it takes to melt these kernels of tension. Others respond to more vigorous pressure. If you do apply strong pressure, be sure to start gently and increase your pressure very gradually. Myotherapists tend to work firmly, applying intense pressure on one area for several minutes at a time. It is important to breathe deeply and focus "through the pain" until it dissolves. If you can't take the pain, lighten up the pressure gradually rather than suddenly pulling away. If you plan to self-treat, we recommend that you make at least one visit to a myotherapist so you can experience the techniques. Several books on myotherapy are listed in the Sources and Suggested Readings section.

- Using the fingertips of your index and middle fingers, press against the muscles over the bones surrounding the eye until you discover a sensitive spot—an area that causes

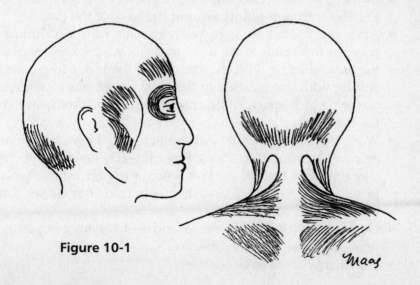

Figure 10-1

you some pain or discomfort when you press on it. When you do, apply pressure for 5 seconds and then release. Do this for both eyes.

- After you complete both eyes, close your eyes if you have not already. Using three or four fingers on each hand, raise the eyebrows as high as possible and hold for 5 seconds. Then push down on the eyebrows for 5 seconds and release. Repeat this sequence three times.
- With your eyes still closed, move your eyes ("look") to the left, right, up, and down. Relax for a moment and then repeat.
- Now explore for trigger points on your nose and apply pressure when you find a sensitive spot.
- Using two fingers on each side of the nose, stretch the muscles by pulling them toward the cheeks. If you have sinus congestion, this work on your nose may relieve all the pressure and cause your nose to run.
- Now explore for trigger points in your cheeks and apply pressure as needed.
- Complete work on the cheeks by using two fingers to stretch the cheeks toward the side.
- At the outside edge of your eyes, apply pressure with your two fingers every $1/2$ inch as you look for trigger points.
- Moving to your ears, again press every $1/2$ inch as you search for trigger points around the back of the ear.
- After you finish both ears, use a knuckle-rolling technique on your forehead. Make a fist and roll your knuckles over the area, starting with the knuckle of the index finger and ending with the knuckle of the little finger. Start each roll about $1/2$ inch apart. After every three or four rolls, stretch the forehead.
- Work the trigger points and the temples, where headache pain is often located. Using three fingers, make small circles on the scalp. When you reach a trigger point, apply pressure for 5 seconds and then continue your circles. Do both sides of your head.
- Go to the back of your head and feel for trigger points; press on those that are sensitive.
- Repeat any areas as needed.

MYOTHERAPY AND TEMPOROMANDIBULAR JOINT SYNDROME

Many myotherapists have excellent success in treating temporo-mandibular joint (TMJ) syndrome and its associated headache. Treatment typically includes locating trigger points in the jaw area and on the back of the head and neck, the upper back, and the shoulders. Use of the elbow is recommended for the back and shoulders; therefore, a myotherapist or a friend who has learned the techniques will have to treat these spots for you. The fingers are used to treat points in the mouth, especially on the gums.

Researchers and physicians are not certain exactly why myo-therapy works. Yet many people attest to the fact that it is an effective method of pain relief for headache and TMJ, with its associated head pain.

OSTEOPATHY

Osteopathy is a philosophy of health care based on the concepts that the human body and its functions, mind, and spirit are interdependent; that the body tends to be self-regulating and self-healing when faced with disease; and that health depends on the unimpaired flow of neural, circulatory, and nutritional forces throughout the body. Osteopathic manipulation is a very successful treatment of both tension headaches and migraines, especially those accompanied by pain and stiffness in the neck, and headaches associated with whiplash, poor posture, sinus-itis, TMJ syndrome, arthritis, and many other causes.

Osteopaths receive the same medical training as their allo-pathic (M.D.) colleagues, with the addition of manual skills as part of their general medical or specialty training. Many osteo-paths choose osteopathic school not only because of its compre-hensive medical training but also because of its holistic, hands-on approach. After completing medical school and postgraduate training, osteopaths choose to specialize in any area of medicine, from pediatrics to surgical subspecialties. Most osteopaths are primary caregivers, fully integrated into the clinic and hospital health network with their M.D. colleagues. Many osteopaths continue to develop their manipulative skills throughout their careers, where they use them as their primary focus or integrate osteopathy into family practice. Many combine homeopathy, acupuncture, and other fields of natural medicine in their practices.

HOW DOES OSTEOPATHY WORK?

Successful osteopathic treatment depends on locating the specific areas of your musculoskeletal system or other parts of the body that need adjustment and on your ability to maintain alignment later by postural awareness and exercise. A misalignment in your pelvic area, for example, may affect your lower back, which affects your upper back, which affects your neck and may cause headache pain. Thus, the thorough examinations osteopaths perform are necessary in order to pinpoint the cause of your pain, including the possibility of other medical problems.

OSTEOPATHIC MANIPULATION AND HEADACHE PAIN

Osteopathic *manipulations* are movements generally performed by an osteopathic physician on the bones, joints, muscles, and fascia (membranes that support or cover the muscles), sometimes with the active assistance of the recipient. It is not typically a treatment you can give yourself, although many osteopaths recommend exercises and some teach manipulations you can do once you have been diagnosed. Specific movements to stretch, loosen, strengthen, and coordinate body motions for stress and pain relief are recommended. The sample balance movements in Chapter 7 are just a few of the possibilities; others can be seen on the balance movements videotape referred to in Appendix II. Also see the box on page 159 for an osteopathic approach to relief of headache related to TMJ syndrome.

Osteopathic manipulation is designed to increase range of motion, improve joint mobility and alignment, stimulate body functions, and increase circulation. Osteopaths work toward this goal using as few manipulations and treatments as are necessary so as not to overstretch the ligaments that hold the bones together. The goal is to treat with minimum force for maximum effect. Osteopaths focus not so much on structure as they do on functional ability. Often individuals have a structural misalign-

EIGHT STEPS TO RELIEF OF TEMPOROMANDIBULAR JOINT SYNDROME

1. Gently massage down your cheeks and let your jaw fall open in a relaxed position that responds to the downward guidance of your fingers.

2. Shake your head gently from side to side so your jaw swings freely, and vocalize "uh" as you do so, to relax your tongue and palate.

3. Yawn widely, gapping the joint to its maximum comfort.

4. Move your jaw from side to side and back and forth as much as is comfortable.

5. Let your jaw hang open in a relaxed position throughout the day.

6. Stand in front of a mirror and practice opening and shutting your mouth slowly while keeping your front teeth aligned.

7. Relax when chewing.

8. Practice self-talk: repeat to yourself each night before you go to sleep, "My jaw is relaxed all night long."

ment that is not the cause of their pain. If the limb or joint moves well and does not hinder full function, the area may not need aggressive treatment.

During your first visit to an osteopath (see Appendix I for help in finding an osteopath), you will likely be asked to give a detailed medical history and report any accidents or falls you have experienced since childhood, as well as significant emotional traumas or wounds. The medical evaluation typically includes a neurologic, orthopedic, and structural examination and palpation (examining by touch) of your spine and related structures to locate any tender points and to evaluate posture and movement.

So that the osteopath can see how well your muscles and bones work together, you may be asked to bend forward and to the sides, to lift your knees, and do other simple movements. This part of the examination usually begins with you in the standing position to be sure that the pelvis and the base of your spine are balanced and symmetrical. Frequently, the area that is causing the pain is distant from the site that hurts. The osteopath also will check the movement of key joints to determine their function and structure.

The osteopath may order x-rays to rule out any physical disorder if your symptoms or history indicate a possible abnormality of your bones, muscles, or tendons, or if he or she suspects a problem that would prevent the use of certain manipulations. Generally, however, osteopaths resort to radiographs and tests only when absolutely necessary. Osteopaths usually can diagnose and frequently relieve the pain within the first or second visit using palpation and correction, thus saving patients time, money, and suffering. Some patients need to return several times a week or once a week for 1 or 2 months.

Many osteopaths are also trained to give specialized injection therapy such as trigger-point treatment. Trigger-point injections are very helpful for headaches caused by tiny, extremely tender knots in muscles that shoot pain to the head. Injection with a homeopathic solution, such as arnica or St. John's wort prepared solely for this purpose usually, but not always, provides immediate relief without adverse effects. Some patients describe the results as "miraculous." Injection of local anesthesia, which can cause side effects as well as be more painful and less long lasting, are sometimes used (see Lidocaine, in Chapter 14).

Osteopaths may write a prescription for pain medications, use herbal medicines, recommend exercise and nutritional strategies, or make referrals to physical therapists and other practitioners. The treatment you receive will depend on the results of your diagnosis.

PHYSICAL THERAPY

Many people think physical therapists work only with accident victims or stroke patients. They picture them in hospitals or rehabilitation centers surrounded by exercise equipment and wheelchairs. The truth is, physical therapists treat many different disorders, including headaches. More and more they are incorporating natural therapies into their practices.

When you go to a physical therapist, you will likely see specialized exercise equipment and traction bars, but these are only a part of a therapy program. Physical therapists are trained to evaluate muscles, bones, and joints and to combine active exercise programs with electrical, ultrasound, and temperature therapies to treat various conditions.

HOW PHYSICAL THERAPY WORKS

Physical therapy consists of various therapeutic techniques designed to strengthen muscles, improve range of motion, increase body awareness, and ultimately to relieve and prevent pain. Choose a physical therapist who will teach you how to take charge of your pain and your therapy. The therapist's goal should be to make you an ex-client—and as pain free as possible. The commitment must come from you.

PHYSICAL THERAPY FOR HEADACHE

Your doctor may refer you to a physical therapist—a practice that is necessary in some states in order for insurance to cover the therapist's costs—or you may select one yourself.

At the first visit, the physical therapist takes a medical history and consults with the patient's physician if necessary. Then he or she and the patient draw up a treatment plan. This may involve manual manipulation of the neck, shoulders, and head; exercises to strength the neck and back; traction in the case of neck injuries; and possibly the use of TENS in cases of chronic pain (discussed later in this chapter). Many physical therapists are trained in various therapies, and they can show you how to treat yourself through application of hot and cold packs, reflexology, and acupressure, among other techniques.

PHYSICAL THERAPY YOU CAN PERFORM

One very important treatment approach for tension headaches and headaches associated with whiplash or other trauma in that area is posture cueing. Posture cueing is a periodic reminder to yourself to be aware of your posture and to correct it with a simple procedure.

For example, the trapezoid muscles that pull the shoulders up toward your ears have many trigger points that refer pain to the head. An easy routine can eliminate this pain. Throughout the day, take a moment to note if your shoulders are tense and hunched, a common posture for people who sit for long periods at a desk or computer. Frequently take a moment to note any tension in your shoulders and consciously lower them to a relaxed position. Another way to relax your shoulders is to do shoulder rolls. Stand with your arms hanging loosely at your sides. Make a big circle with your shoulders by lifting your shoulders toward your ears. Then push your shoulders forward, down, and back, and up again in a big circle. Continue in this circular motion 5 to 10 times, always keeping your arms hanging straight down. Repeat this motion in the other direction. Do this every hour or at lunch and during breaks.

Aerobic exercise—activity that increases oxygen use, such as running, walking, and swimming—is another important part of physical therapy for headache. Exercise flushes tissues with cleansing blood and oxygen and removes metabolic by-products. Physical therapists often recommend exercise programs suited to an individual's physical condition and needs.

SWEDISH MASSAGE

Swedish massage was developed about 150 years ago by Peter Ling of Sweden primarily as a medical treatment. It incorporates several basic strokes that are used on the soft tissues of the body to bring about release of muscle tension and pain, including headache pain. Unlike Oriental massage (see Chapter 9), Swedish massage therapists use oils and work directly on the unclothed body and focus their massage movements toward the heart.

HOW DOES SWEDISH MASSAGE WORK?

In addition to the relaxation benefits of Swedish massage, it increases circulation, improves functioning of sweat glands, nourishes and rejuvenates the skin, and stimulates the flow of nutrients to the cells as it releases toxins from underlying fatty tissue. At the same time, it contributes to more flexible joints, tendons, and muscles. If you have headache associated with gastrointestinal problems such as constipation or poor digestion, massage of the abdomen can help relieve these conditions.

SWEDISH MASSAGE FOR HEADACHES

Swedish masseurs recommend and perform full-body massage because of the overall benefits it provides. However, they can focus on areas that need particular attention, specifically the head, neck, and shoulders in cases of headache and TMJ, and on the abdomen for headache associated with digestive problems. Swedish massage involves long, deep strokes that work best when you are a relaxed recipient. If possible, have a professional masseur or a friend do the massage. Oriental massage and other pressure-point therapies (Chapter 9) are more geared for self-treatment.

The instructions given here concentrate on the neck, head, and abdomen and are written for the person giving you the massage. Use a massage table, or arrange for your comfort on the floor: towels, blankets, a futon, a sleeping bag, or a thin foam mattress for padding. Some people add a pillow or rolled towel under their knees, neck, or head when they lie face up, or under their ankles, pelvis, or chest when they lie face down. Begin the massage lying face up, and feel free to adjust your position for greater comfort as the massage goes on. Choose a spot that allows enough room for your friend to touch and even lean into muscles that need massage. Have coconut, almond, or an herbal massage oil available (see box on page 164), warmed if you like.

Note: Throughout the massage, both you and the recipient should always be in a comfortable position.

Neck

Kneel behind the person's head. Place both hands underneath the neck with your wrists flat on the mat. Knead the neck with your fingertips for several minutes. Here, as throughout the massage, apply only as much pressure as the person finds comfortable. The recipient may have tender areas that require special care. Always use very slow, gentle pressure when you begin to work on any area and gradually build up pressure only if the person is comfortable with it.

HERBAL MASSAGE OILS

Consider one of these herbal massage oils when getting a massage:

- *Jojoba oil:* Use cold-pressed jojoba oil. This odorless oil has anti-inflammatory properties that are destroyed if the oil is heated in processing.

- *St. John's wort oil:* This red oil is good for nerve pain. Mix it in equal proportions with jojoba or aloe vera oil.

Make your own massage oils. For a relaxing combination, mix 1¾ fluid oz. jojoba oil with 10 drops sandalwood oil, 5 drops Roman chamomile, and 2 drops each of coriander and rose. Or you can experiment with jojoba oil and any of the following essential oils: lavender, balm, geranium, orange, tangerine, cedar. Use small amounts: the acids in even common oils, such as citrus, can irritate sensitive skin.

Face

Facial massage requires little if any oil on your fingers. Massage along the neck and sides of the face using gentle circles directed toward the scalp or away from the nose, across the cheeks, and toward the ears. Continue for several minutes. Then place your thumbs or index fingers over the cheekbones and massage gently under the eye sockets and toward the temples.

With your index fingers placed below each eye, make gentle circular strokes around the orbits that move up the outer sides of the eyes toward the top of the head and then down the bridge of the nose.

Using your fingers and thumbs, apply tiny, deep, circular motions on the forehead. This loosens tightness in muscle fibers. Then go to the ears and, beginning with the lobes, continue to gently rub small circles around the outer ear.

If the recipient has headache associated with digestive problems, an abdomen massage may provide relief. (If not, you may skip to the last paragraph of these instructions.) Place your left hand on top of your right hand and, using light pressure and a circular motion, massage from the pubic area up to just under the bottom of the rib cage and then back down to the pubic area. Repeat 5 to 10 times, increasing the size of the circles slightly to include more of the front abdominal area. You can increase the amount of pressure each time if it is comfortable for the recipient.

Rub your hands together briskly to warm them, place your open palms over the recipient's eyes or on the sides of his or her head, and hold them there gently for 10 to 20 seconds as a quiet way to complete your massage.

TRANSCUTANEOUS ELECTRICAL NERVE STIMULATION

TENS for headache pain involves placing small electrodes directly on acupuncture or trigger points on the head and neck. These electrodes emit a pulsating electrical stimulus to the nerves underneath them. TENS can be provided continuously through a small, portable electrical charger worn on a belt. It is a safe and effective alternative to drug therapy that can be used by most people who suffer with chronic headache pain. The only side effect is that occasionally the electrodes can irritate sensitive skin. Individuals with a pacemaker need to check with their physician before using TENS, as the frequencies emitted by the unit may interfere with pacemaker function.

HOW DOES TRANSCUTANEOUS ELECTRICAL NERVE STIMULATION WORK?

Exactly how TENS relieves pain is not clear. Experts believe the stimulation may help release the body's own pain relievers (endorphins and enkephalins), or it may shut off the relay of pain sensations, similar to the theory behind acupuncture's effectiveness. Regardless of the reason, TENS relieves a significant amount of headache pain for a period of time for many individuals who have chronic headache pain.

TRANSCUTANEOUS ELECTRICAL NERVE STIMULATION FOR HEADACHE

A physician must prescribe TENS for you, and the units are typically dispensed and explained by a physical therapist or nurse, who then monitors your progress. Depending on the severity and extent of your headache, it may take several days or weeks before you notice a substantial improvement. Be patient. Because you can wear the TENS unit at all times, you have the ability to turn it on and off when you need it and control the amount of stimulation. More than half of people with chronic pain have a good response to TENS. After about 1 year of use, however, the initial good results decrease to about 30 percent as the nervous system develops a higher tolerance for the stimulation and lets the pain messages go through. TENS works best when combined with natural therapies such as biofeedback and other relaxation techniques, as well as life-style changes. Many people who use TENS find that it gives them enough time and relief to allow them to pursue other therapies—such as biofeedback and hypnosis—that they can use when TENS begins to lose its effectiveness.

SYNAPTIC ELECTRONIC ACTIVATION

Synaptic Electronic Activation (SEA) is a high-frequency wave generator, similar in appearance to a TENS unit, that offers people with headache a new, noninvasive way to treat their pain. The SEA unit can provide long-term pain relief for people with chronic pain and has been approved by most insurance companies for this use.

Like a TENS unit, a SEA device has electrodes that are placed on the body to deliver stimulation to the nerves. Several differences between TENS and SEA, however, are that SEA can deliver the stimulation at a much higher frequency than does TENS (180 Hz, compared with up to 30,000 Hz with SEA), and you have a handheld remote control that allows you to increase or decrease the intensity of treatment as needed. Also, skin irritation is a minor problem with SEA because it uses special electrode pads that have hypoallergenic adhesive.

HOW DOES SEA WORK?

Pain signals travel along the nerve cell bodies as waves and are translated into chemical neurotransmitters once they reach the end, or synapse, of a nerve. These neurotransmitters move across the synapse and carry the pain message to the next nerve cell, and so on. The SEA unit helps eliminate pain by modifying the neurotransmitters and thus disrupting the pain signals.

Blood samples taken before and after treatment with SEA show that neurotransmitter secretion levels, such as endorphins (the body's natural pain killers), serotonin, and epinephrine, change and remain modified 24 hours and longer after treatment. In addition to modifying pain transmission, nerve stimulation with SEA also promotes production of endorphins.

SEA FOR HEADACHE

Like a TENS unit, a SEA device must be prescribed by your doctor. She or her staff will explain how the unit works and monitor your progress. To treat headache, two to four electrodes are placed on either side of the painful area. Once the device is turned on, it emits two signals that you can control to relieve your pain. The intensity control button allows you to increase or decrease the impulses sent to your nerves. You can turn up the intensity until you feel a slight tingling at the electrode sites. The second adjustment is to the bias control, which lets you change the intensity of the tingling. The goal during treatment is to maintain a constant comfortable signal from the SEA device to the nerves by adjusting the bias control from zero to its maximum level. After you reach the maximum bias amount at one intensity level, you will increase the intensity level by one increment and then begin to increase the bias at the new intensity level. Depending on the severity and duration of your headache pain, you may start with three 15- to 20-minute sessions per week and decrease them as needed.

All of the therapies explained in this chapter help prevent and treat headache pain using physical healing techniques, yet each one differs in how it approaches that goal. We hope the diverse options offered here provide something for everyone and that whichever therapies you choose, they provide you with headache pain relief.

11

DIET AND NUTRITION

Your diet very likely has both a direct and indirect effect on your headaches. Consuming substances such as caffeine, monosodium glutamate (MSG), nitrates and nitrites (found in processed meats), and tyramine (in meats, peanuts, and other foods) can cause headaches in sensitive individuals. These dietary culprits frequently have an immediate impact on your headache. Other substances have a delayed effect, such as alcohol, which causes dehydration headaches, or eating lots of junk food, which depletes magnesium and other nutrients needed for proper muscle tone. An imbalance of magnesium can cause muscle tension headache.

Diet affects head pain through several mechanisms. One is that headaches occur in people who are genetically or environmentally sensitive to one or more naturally occurring chemicals, such as caffeine and tyramines, or to food additives that are in many foods and beverages. The intensity and frequency of the headaches depend on how sensitive the person is to the chemicals. A person may be sensitive to more than one food, and the foods do not need to be chemically similar in order to cause a reaction. Another theory suggests that people who get headaches have an allergy to some foods that their body perceives as a foreign substance, or *antigen*. Other food-related causes of headaches include vitamin deficiencies, skipped meals, and poor nutrition, all of which place stress on the body's function and organ systems.

THE HEALTHIEST EATING PLAN

Proper nutrition is a major preventive measure against headache, as well as many diseases, including the three leading killers—heart disease, stroke, and cancer. At the same time, balanced, healthy eating will boost general health and well-being and help you reduce or eliminate headache pain associated with common medical conditions, such as constipation, hormone fluctuations, and hypoglycemia (low blood sugar levels).

Ideally, a whole-grain, whole-bean, plant-based diet that avoids processed foods is best. You can meet all your nutritional needs if you eat a wide variety of fresh vegetables, a large salad daily (use vinegar-based dressings sparingly or not at all), and make most of your meals from whole foods—foods you purchase in their original form, rather than those that are processed, precooked, and packaged for microwave convenience. Whole foods come without the chemical additives, and nutritional value is not lost to processing. If you are not used to cooking with whole foods, you might take some cooking classes, exchange recipes with friends, or consult some of the many excellent cookbooks that are available (see Sources and Suggested Readings for this section).

As a rough general guideline, the daily diet of an active adult should include the following:

- 2–4 cups whole grains (one piece of bread is $^1/_4$ to $^1/_2$ cup)
- $^1/_2$–1 cup legumes (beans, including soy)
- 4–6 cups dark green leafy and yellow vegetables
- $^1/_2$–1 cup starchy vegetables, like potatoes
- 0–2 pieces of fruit
- 1–3 tbsp. cold-pressed oil
- 1–3 tbsp. sea vegetables or blue-green algae, nutritional yeast

Figure 11-1 represents this eating plan. This is a modification of the food pyramid formulated by the U.S. Department of Agriculture, whose pyramid has a section for meat and dairy products and lacks the healthy oils and algae foods that provide all your nutrient requirements without the need for food supplements. The pyramid shown here is based on the plan approved by the Physicians Committee for Responsible Medicine and other health organizations as the healthiest eating plan not only for overall health but for prevention of headache and diseases such as cancer, heart disease, diabetes, stroke, hypertension, kidney disease, and many others. We have added other categories to ensure adequate intake of antioxidants (specific vitamins, minerals, and other nutrients which, among other things, fight cell-damaging agents called free radicals and also strengthen the immune system) and essential fatty acids, which are explained later in this chapter.

The following suggestions round out the guidelines given above. You may have to adjust some of them to reflect any medical problems you have or medications you may be taking.

- If you do not have access to a wide variety of whole foods, choose the least refined and processed foods that you can, and try to avoid chemical additives especially.
- Consume minimal or no animal products—meat, dairy, and fish—for overall health reasons as well as for the chemicals that are concentrated in these foods that may be triggering your headache pain. For dairy items in particular, many people have an undetected allergy or intolerance to milk products. (Indeed, in many cases of food allergy, the same foods we crave are the very ones to which we are allergic.) Dairy foods also are mucus-forming, and many experts believe they are a factor in sinusitis (see Chapter 5).
- Choose whole, unrefined grains. Brown rice, wheat, corn, beans, barley, rye, millet, and buckwheat are some of the most common choices. We suggest you try some unusual and tasty grains as well, such as quinoa, spelt, and kamut.
- Select fresh, organic vegetables and fruits as the majority of your diet whenever possible, as well as blue-green algae, and a variety of mushrooms and sea vegetables (such as nori, agar, kombu, wakame, kelp, and hijiki—all available in Oriental groceries and health-food stores), which are rich in vitamins and protein.

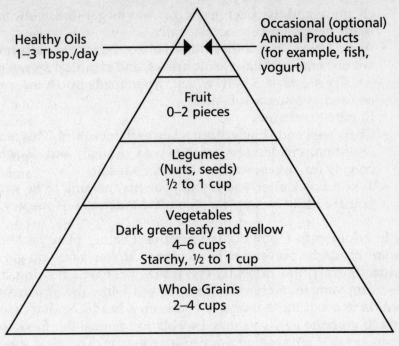

Healthy Oils
1–3 Tbsp./day

Occasional (optional)
Animal Products
(for example, fish,
yogurt)

Fruit
0–2 pieces

Legumes
(Nuts, seeds)
½ to 1 cup

Vegetables
Dark green leafy and yellow
4–6 cups
Starchy, ½ to 1 cup

Whole Grains
2–4 cups

Figure 11-1

- Always wash fruits and vegetables well, especially if they are not organic. Washing helps remove external contaminants, including parasites. Nonorganic produce frequently contains pesticides in the food flesh, and these cannot be washed away.
- When choosing healthy oils, flax, safflower, and sunflower oils are best as they contain significant amounts of essential fatty acids. Do not use in cooking. Olive oil is also excellent, but it contains less fatty acids than the other three mentioned. Sesame and coconut oils are the most stable oils for cooking.
- Use sea salt, miso, soy sauce (all high in sodium, use sparingly), instead of table salt, which lacks more complex nutrition. To reduce salt intake, explore fresh or dried herbs, such as basil, oregano, garlic, thyme, and dill, to replace salt when you cook. Do not use MSG, seasonings with

chemical additives, refined sugar, or vinegar (too acidic for many people) except occasionally.

- Avoid fried and other high-fat foods, sugar, alcohol, sweets, enriched dairy, soft drinks, and chemical sweeteners. Try stevia—an herb which, when made into a tea, can be used as a sugar substitute.
- Eliminate caffeine.
- Chew well and slowly; appreciate each mouthful. This aids digestion, creates less tendency to overeat, and lessens craving for sweets and liquids after a meal.
- Take a break after you finish your first helping to be sure you are really hungry for seconds. Moderation is the key.

In addition to following the healthiest eating plan, another part of headache prevention is avoidance. If you *know* you get a headache every time or nearly every time you have a hot dog, an ice-cream sundae, a chocolate bar, or red wine, the best treatment is to avoid these foods. If you keep a headache diary (see sample on page 18), you may be able to identify the foods or beverages that are causing your headache pain. The good news about chocolate is that white chocolate may not cause the same response as regular chocolate!

If you *suspect* certain food items are causing your headaches but cannot definitely identify them, you can use an elimination diet (explained below) to pinpoint the culprit foods.

HEADACHE, DIET, HORMONES, AND HYPOGLYCEMIA

The healthiest eating plan, outlined above, can help women reduce the headaches and other side effects of hormone fluctuations that are associated with the menstrual cycle (known as premenstrual syndrome [PMS]), use of oral contraceptives, and menopause. Increased intake of complex carbohydrates (pasta, grains, potatoes, bread, vegetables), for example, helps regulate mood swings that commonly occur when hormone levels change. Reduced salt intake, especially the week before the menstrual cycle starts, can help control the bloating and headaches that frequently result from increased pressure caused by water retention. Soy-based foods are most helpful in balancing female hormone levels and can relieve headaches associated with PMS, especially when eaten as a replacement for meat.

Skipping meals can lower blood sugar levels (hypoglycemia) and trigger a hunger headache or a migraine in some individuals. Eating five or six small meals or planned snacks during the day can help keep blood sugar levels relatively even. This doesn't mean you will eat more; you will simply spread the amount you usually eat over the day. Keep a supply of nuts, seeds, sea and fresh vegetables, dried fruits, or whole-grain crackers handy for snacking.

HEADACHES, DIET, AND CONSTIPATION

Headache often accompanies constipation, and one of the best natural ways to prevent and eliminate both of these conditions is with a diet that is naturally high in fiber, as is the one above. Forget drugstore laxatives; if you follow a healthy diet and drink at least eight glasses of liquid a day, you probably won't need them. Liquid is essential: too little makes it difficult for fiber to leave the intestines and can make constipation worse. Regular exercise also is important, as it helps keep the intestines active and healthy. If constipation is still a problem, you can try 1 tsp. psyllium seeds or hulls in 1 cup of water, followed by 1 or more cups of water. Also helpful are 2,000 mg of vitamin C every few hours or 1 tbsp. flax seed or hemp oil taken in one swallow.

SWITCHING TO THE HEALTHIEST EATING PLAN

We realize that these nutritional recommendations may represent a significantly different diet than the one you currently follow. Make your changes gradually. Consider lean meat, chicken, and fish to be a condiment: reduce your intake to 2 to 4 oz. a day instead of the 8 oz. or more you may be consuming now. As you eliminate meat and dairy products, gradually try new foods; dozens of suggestions and hundreds of recipes can be found in the books in Sources and Suggested Readings.

Your new eating plan will be easier when you have support and easily accessible, current information. If you need help in choosing a nutrition plan, seek a nutritionist, osteopath, or naturopath knowledgeable about whole foods. See Appendix I for organizations that can help you find a nutritionist or answer your questions about diet. Hospital dietitians typically do not receive training in whole-food or vegetarian diets.

ELIMINATION DIET PLAN

Food intolerance and allergy have a major role in causing migraines. In a well-controlled study conducted at the Hospital for Sick Children in London, Dr. Joseph Egger studied the effects of food intolerance on 88 children aged 3 to 18 who had severe migraines. Once the children eliminated certain "culprit" foods from their diet, 93 percent recovered completely from headache within 3 weeks. The top seven foods were cow's milk (the cause in 30 percent of cases), eggs (27 percent), chocolate (25 percent), oranges (24 percent), wheat (24 percent), cheese (15 percent), and tomatoes (15 percent). Eighty percent of children reacted to more than one food. Research indicates that these and other foods have a similar role in adult migraines.

If you have used the headache diary (see page 18) and have not yet determined if food is at the root of your headache pain, try the elimination diet plan. This plan can take several months to complete, but in the end, you will likely know which food(s) to avoid to prevent or reduce your migraine attacks. A sample elimination diet plan appears below. If you routinely drink caffeine beverages or take medications that contain caffeine, you need to slowly taper off of them before you start this plan. In general, take 3 days for every one cup of coffee or cola you drink per day. If you drink three cups per day, for example, it will take you 9 days to completely eliminate the beverage to prevent withdrawal headache. Base your withdrawal time on 50 to 100 mg less of caffeine every 3 days. See Table 11-1 on page 175 for the caffeine content of various substances.

- Once you have eliminated caffeine completely for at least 1 week, avoid all foods listed in the box on page 176 for 10 to 30 days. During this "rest" period, your body will become even more sensitive to whatever food(s) may be triggering your pain.
- Between days 5 and 14 of the elimination diet, your headache and other symptoms should be nearly or totally gone,

TABLE 11-1.
Caffeine Content of Common Foods and Drugs (in mg)

Beverages (6 oz.)	Caffeine Content	OTC Drugs*	Caffeine Content
Drip coffee	120–150	Dexatrim	200
Percolated coffee	80–110	Vivarin	200
Instant coffee	60–100	NoDoz	100
Decaffeinated coffee	3–10	Aqua-Ban	100
Tea, black or green	30–60	Cafergot	100
Colas	30–65	Excedrin	65
Chocolate milk	10–15	Vanquish	33
		Midol	32

*Over-the-counter drugs; amount of caffeine per regular-strength tablet.

if food is the immediate cause of your headache pain. If you still have pain, you may need to eliminate more foods from your diet, or your headache may not be caused by food.

- Once your headaches disappear or decrease substantially, begin to add items back to your diet. Add one at a time, preferably one new item every 2 days, at one or two meals.
- If you react to a reintroduced food, the symptoms will be stronger than they were before you went on the elimination diet. Once you react to an item, omit the food from your diet again and wait 2 days before you introduce another new food. In most cases, people will respond within 48 hours of eating an introduced food if they are sensitive to it.
- Keep a detailed record of each food you introduce—when introduced and any reactions you have to it. It's important to keep this record, as it is very possible that more than one food is causing your headache.
- If you have already reacted once to a reintroduced food and want to verify that it is causing a reaction, you can reintroduce it a second time. However, allow at least 1 week to pass between the times you add the item to your diet. If you react a second time, eliminate this food from your diet completely.

FOODS THAT CAN TRIGGER HEADACHE

Alcohol*: especially red wine, champagne, and dark liquors
Aspartame (NutraSweet)
Avocados
Bananas
Beans (selected varieties only: lima, fava, navy, broad)
Bread products containing yeast, including sourdough breads
Caffeine (coffee, tea, colas, headache medications)
Cheese* (except cottage, American, and cream cheese)
Chocolate*
Citrus fruits and juices (orange, lemon, lime, grapefruit)
Cold foods
Figs (canned)
Herring*
Meats—processed and cured (bologna, hot dogs, salami, bacon, sausage, pepperoni)
Monosodium glutamate (MSG)
Nuts and nut butters, including peanuts* and peanut butter
Onions
Organ meats*
Pea pods
Pineapple and its juice
Raisins
Red plums
Sauerkraut*
Sour cream
Tomatoes (and other nightshades such as potatoes, eggplant, and peppers)
Wheat
Yogurt

Note: The foods listed above commonly trigger headache pain. *Any* food to which you are sensitive, however, can cause headache.

*Contain tyramine, an amino acid that triggers headache in some individuals.

Between 20 and 25 percent of people who have migraine headaches get substantial relief when they follow a tyramine-free diet. Foods that contain this naturally appearing amino acid are marked with an asterisk (*) in the box on page 176.

If the elimination diet is frustrating or not helpful to you, we recommend you consult allergy-testing laboratories and ask for a test called an ELISA ACT, such as that offered by Serammune Physicians Lab (see Appendix I for this and other allergy-testing laboratories). This test covers hundreds of substances, including food additives, environmental chemicals, common foods, and spices and can also identify delayed allergic reactions—those which can take up to several weeks to cause symptoms. Along with the test results you also receive a detailed explanation and guidebook on how to eliminate the foods that affect you.

NUTRITIONAL SUPPLEMENTS AS TREATMENT

A deficiency of some vitamins and minerals can cause headache. Before you start any type of supplement program, however, talk with a nutritionist, dietitian, naturopath, or other professional who is knowledgeable about nutrition for recommendations on supplementation. If you or your practitioner suspect a vitamin or mineral deficiency, consider having your blood analyzed. Some laboratories conduct detailed analyses of blood nutrient levels. Although these tests are controversial, it is likely that individualized nutritional supplement programs based on analysis of blood nutrient levels will become much more widely used. Blood-nutrient analyses are usually expensive, but some insurance companies cover the cost when they are ordered by a physician.

Many patients with headache and symptoms associated with PMS and fatigue get pain relief with daily use of a balanced, high-dose multiple vitamin. In addition to recommending a daily multiple vitamin, some practitioners recommend specific, individual vitamin or mineral supplements as treatment for acute headache.

The vitamins and minerals described in the sections below can help relieve headache pain. To help you determine how much of a particular nutrient you are consuming now, the Recommended Daily Allowance (RDA) for the vitamins and minerals and some common foods that contain them are listed. RDA values are considered to be the *minimum* required to avoid deficiency conditions. If you are already deficient, RDA amounts are not adequate to fulfill your needs, especially if the reasons for the deficiency—such as poor diet, disease, or malabsorption—remain.

Also included here is information on immune-system boosters (see the box on page 184). The immune system is responsible for the body's general health, and both good nutrition and life style play major roles in maintaining the body's defense against disease and symptoms associated with them, such as headache.

The "players" in the immune system include white blood cells, antibodies, and the adrenal gland, liver, spleen, thymus, and skin. Some of the things that inhibit optimal functioning of the immune system are unmanaged stress, obesity, alcohol, insufficient sleep, and poor nutrition, especially intake of fat and simple sugars. To keep your immune system functioning at its best, life-style modifications in these areas need to be made. You also can boost your immune system by taking certain vitamins, minerals, and herbs (see box on page 184). See a knowledgeable health-care practitioner to help you devise a supplemental plan to suit your needs.

B VITAMINS: FOLIC ACID, NIACIN, B_6, AND B_{12}

B vitamins should be taken together, as they work cooperatively. A deficiency of folic acid, niacin (vitamin B_3), or B_6 has been linked to headache pain. Folic acid is water-soluble, which means it is found in the watery part of foods, does not need fat to be absorbed by the body, and dissolves in blood. Unlike fat-soluble vitamins, which are stored in the body, most folic acid is excreted in the urine and needs to be replaced often. The RDAs for folic acid are as follows: 200 mcg for males 15 years and older; 180 mcg for females 15 years and older; 400 and 260 to 280 mcg for pregnant and lactating females, respectively.

A niacin deficiency (the term commonly used to refer to the two forms of vitamin B_3—nicotinic acid and nicotinamide) can occur when you eat very little protein. The RDA for niacin is 19 mg for men 19 to 50 years and 15 mg for older men; for women, 15 mg for those 19 to 50 years, 17 mg and 20 mg for those who are pregnant or lactating, respectively, and 13 mg for older women. To treat acute headache pain, take 50 to 200 mg of nicotinamide three times per day, as the nicotinic acid form causes temporary flushing, tingling in the arms and legs, burning, and itching in some individuals. (Check the label on your multivitamin bottle.)

Vitamin B_6, pyridoxine, is a necessary component in raising serotonin levels, which in turn increase the pain threshold. Supplements of this vitamin are used by people with stress, headache, insomnia, and fatigue. Vitamin B_6 also is a natural diuretic and is useful in treating symptoms related to PMS, especially water retention and headache.

The RDA for adults of B_6 is 10 to 15 mg per day. Much of this vitamin is lost during cooking and processing. One of the richest sources is wheat germ, and a good level is available in whole grains, soybeans and other dried beans, peanuts, walnuts, bananas, prunes, and potatoes.

Although headache is not generally associated with a deficiency of vitamin B_{12}, investigations involving vitamin B_{12} show that it can block adverse reactions to sulfites and other common food additives that cause headache in many people. It also can relieve chronic pain. Injections of 1,000 mcg of B_{12} into the muscle is an effective way to take this vitamin. Sublingual supplements (tablets that dissolve under the tongue) are taken at higher doses to allow for absorption loss.

TABLE 11-2.
Amount of Niacin Equivalent* in Chosen Foods

Food	Niacin (mg)	Tryptophan (mg)	Niacin Equivalent (mg)
Chicken, ½ breast	15.5	205	21.5
Salmon, 3 oz.	6.8	200	9.6
Peanut butter, 2 tbsp.	4.8	305	6.2
Peas, green, 1 cup	2.7	66	4.5
Potato, medium	2.7	33	3.6
Brewer's yeast, 1 tbsp.	3.0	429	3.6

*Although niacin is a vitamin, it is also produced in the body when it teams up with the amino acid tryptophan. The conversion of tryptophan to niacin provides the body with more than 50% of its daily requirement of niacin.

To see how you fare with folic acid and niacin intake, see Tables 11-2 and 11-3 for some foods high in these vitamins.

CHOLINE

Supplementation with choline, a micronutrient, may be helpful in reducing cluster headache pain. Some people with cluster headache also have been found to have low levels of this nutrient.

The body manufactures choline with the help of vitamin B_{12}, folic acid, and methionine, an amino acid. Choline helps prevent fat build-up in the liver and is necessary for normal nerve and brain function. No RDA has been established for choline. A well-balanced diet for adults contains approximately 400 to 900 mg of choline, most of which comes from eggs, liver, lean meat, brewer's yeast, soybeans, peanuts, and green peas. If your diet lacks foods rich in choline and folic acid (see Table 11-3), you

TABLE 11-3.
Amount of Folic Acid in Chosen Foods

Food	Folic Acid (mcg)
Brewer's yeast, 1 tbsp.	313
Bulgur, cooked, ⅔ cup	158
Okra, cooked, ½ cup	134
Kidney beans, red, cooked, ½ cup	114
Spinach, raw, 1 cup	106
Orange juice, 6 oz.	102
Soybeans, cooked, ½ cup	100
Lettuce, romaine, 1 cup	98
Beets, cooked, ½ cup	66
Avocado, ½ medium	59
Broccoli, cooked, ½ cup	44
Wheat germ, 2 tbsp.	40
Beans, red, cooked, ½ cup	34
Banana, 1 medium	33
Brussels sprouts, cooked, ½ cup	28
Bread, wheat, 1 slice	16

may want to add brewer's yeast to your diet. Brewer's yeast can be added to soups, stews, or sprinkled on popcorn. Start with $^1/_4$ tsp., as many people are sensitive to this food.

COPPER, ZINC, AND IRON

When there is not enough copper in the diet, headache pain can be the result. Copper is involved in the metabolism of serotonin, tyramine, and catecholamines, all substances that affect the nerves and blood vessels in the brain. The RDA is 1.5 to 3.0 mg for adults of both sexes.

The balance among iron, zinc, and copper is important (see Table 11.5) for proper absorption of copper; thus, you need to watch your intake of these minerals as well. Because copper can rise to toxic levels, we recommend that you undergo a blood analysis of your mineral levels before starting copper supplementation. The RDA for zinc is 15 mg for adult men and 12 mg for adult women. Iron deficiency is common, especially among women of childbearing age. The RDAs are as follows: men 19 years and older, 10 mg; females 11 to 50 years, 15 mg; pregnant females, 30 mg; lactating females, 15 mg; women 51 years and older, 10 mg. The content of copper, zinc, and iron in selected foods is shown in Tables 11-4 and 11-5.

TABLE 11-4.
Copper and Zinc Content in Chosen Foods

Food	Copper (mg)	Zinc (mg)
Oysters, 6 medium	14.2	124.9
Liver, cooked, 3 oz.	2.4	3.3
Avocado, ½	0.5	—
Potato, baked	0.36	0.4
Almonds, ¼ cup	—	1.2
Banana, 1 medium	0.26	—
Spinach, cooked, ½ cup	0.13	0.17
Peas, green, cooked, ½ cup	0.12	—
Bread, whole wheat, 1 slice	0.06	—
Carrots, cooked, ½ cup	0.06	—

TABLE 11-5.
Amount of Iron in Chosen Foods

Food	Iron (mg)
Liver, cooked, 3 oz.	7.5
Oysters, raw, ½ cup	6.6
Apricots, dried, ½ cup	3.6
Molasses, blackstrap, 1 tbsp.	3.2
Ground beef, cooked, 3 oz.	3.0
Raisins, ½ cup	2.6
Navy beans, cooked, ½ cup	2.6
Spinach, cooked, ½ cup	2.4
Lima beans, cooked, ½ cup	2.4
Split peas, cooked, ½ cup	2.1

MAGNESIUM AND CALCIUM

Studies that have used magnesium supplementation for migraine have shown it to be very effective in alleviating or eliminating head pain. Magnesium is considered to be an antistress mineral because one of its functions is to relax the smooth muscles of blood vessels.

Magnesium has a complex relationship with several other important elements in the body, including calcium. Too much calcium in the diet inhibits absorption of magnesium. To maximize the effectiveness of magnesium supplements, take those that are highly absorbable and balanced with an equal amount of calcium. The most readily absorbed magnesium supplements are those chelated (bonded) with amino acids or citrate as opposed to mineral salts such as magnesium bicarbonate and magnesium oxide. For treatment of acute headache, take 200 to 400 mg per hour of calcium and 100 to 200 mg per hour of magnesium for several hours or until substantial relief is achieved.

In 1989, the RDA for magnesium was revised to the following guidelines: adult men, 350 mg daily; adult women, 280 mg; pregnant females, 320 mg; lactating females, 260 to 280 mg. The RDAs for calcium are 1,000 mg daily for men and premeno-

TABLE 11-6.
Magnesium and Calcium Content in Chosen Foods (in mg)

Food	Magnesium Content	Food	Calcium Content
Peanuts, ¼ cup	63	Yogurt, plain, 1 cup	415
Banana, 1 medium	58	Soy milk, fortified, 8 oz.	350
Beet greens, 1 cup	58	Mustard greens, cooked, ½ cup	97
Avocado, ½ medium	56	Orange, 1 medium	54
Peanut butter, 2 tbsp.	56	Broccoli, cooked, ½ cup	50
Cashews, 9 medium	52	Navy beans, cooked, ½ cup	48
Wheat germ, 2 tbsp.	40	Bread, whole wheat, 1 slice	24
Brewer's nutritional yeast, 2 tbsp.	36		
Collard greens, 1 cup	31		
Bread, whole wheat, 1 slice	19		

pausal females and 1,500 mg for postmenopausal women. Food sources of magnesium and calcium are listed in Table 11-6.

OMEGA-3 AND OMEGA-6 FATTY ACIDS

The omega-3 and omega-6 fatty acids (eicosapentaenoic acid, gamma-linolenic acid, and linoleic acid) found in fish oil, borage oil, evening primrose oil, and flaxseed oil, when added to the daily diet, can reduce the severity and frequency of migraine headaches. These fatty acids, which also have anti-inflammatory and anticancer properties, are available as supplements in health-food stores. The recommended dosage is 5 to 20 g per day; take them along with digestive enzymes such as papaya if you have difficulty digesting fats. Flaxseed oil, evening primrose oil, and the more affordable borage oil can "calm down" fluctuating hormones in women with PMS or other hormone-related symptoms.

Diet has a significant impact on overall health and often plays a role in headache pain. A poor eating plan can be a major cause of head pain; however, in this chapter we explained how you

IMMUNE-SYSTEM BOOSTERS

Here are some common immune-system boosters and suggested supplement doses. Consult with your health-care provider for your particular needs. Also refer to Sources and Suggested Readings for more information.

- *Vitamin A:* Helps maintain the skin and mucosal surfaces and enhances the immune system. Take 5,000 IU (international units) daily.

- *Vitamin C:* Stimulates activity of white blood cells and increases the levels of antibodies. Stress causes vitamin C to be excreted excessively in the urine; therefore, supplementation is important for people with stress-related headache. Physicians recommend different dosages, although 500–1,500 mg taken three times daily is common.

- *Beta-carotene:* Protects the epithelial cells (the cells that line the surfaces of organs and the skin) and enhances the immune system. Take 5,000–25,000 IU daily.

- *Zinc:* Necessary for proper function of the thymus and white blood cells. Supplement: 15–30 mg daily. Taking more than 75 mg/day on a regular basis can damage the immune system.

- *Echinacea:* This herb helps increase the production of white blood cells and also helps prevent the spread of viruses. Take 1 tsp. of the extract or tincture in water three times daily for acute viral infections (also see Chapter 13).

- *Licorice:* Studies of this herb suggest it inhibits the growth of human viruses and protects the thymus from cortisone, a stress-related hormone. Licorice root is available in tablets as deglycyrrhizinated licorice, which does not raise blood pressure the way continued use of licorice alone may. Take 760 mg/day.

- *Shiitake mushroom:* This fungus has been used for centuries by the Chinese to increase resistance to infection. Shiitake mushrooms increase production of T-cells and interferon and augments macrophage (cells that engulf foreign particles and assist in general infection resistance) activity. Shiitake can be purchased fresh or dried and added to your recipes. It also is available as a concentrate; take according to label directions.

can make a shift in your diet and supplement it with vitamins and other nutrients to bring about headache pain relief. Although the options presented here may not bring about instant relief, they can provide lifelong solutions once your body has adjusted to the changes.

12

HERBAL MEDICINE AND AROMATHERAPY

Herbal medicine is the use of plant-based remedies for their healing effects on the body. According to the World Health Organization, up to 80 percent of the world's population uses herbal remedies. Most often they are prescribed for everyday ailments, including headache, fever, stomach disorders, and cold symptoms. In this chapter, we look at herbal medicine and a close relative, aromatherapy, and how they can be used to reduce or eliminate headache pain.

HERBAL MEDICINE

Between 30 and 50 percent of all medical doctors in Germany and France routinely use herbal preparations as their main medicines. In the United States, most conventional physicians have not incorporated herbal medicine into their practices. Still, interest in herbalism is mounting among conventional physicians, as people have become concerned about the side effects of drugs and are now more open to a holistic health approach in general. Researchers are now investigating and documenting the claims made for centuries by herbalists from around the globe. While these studies go on, advocates of herbal medicine continue to rely on the wisdom of experience and tradition and seek guidance from those who are knowledgeable in the use of herbs, including herbalists, naturopaths, biochemists, ethnobotanists, and homeopaths.

Many health-care practitioners find plant-based remedies to be highly effective, with far fewer and less dangerous side effects than prescription and over-the-counter drugs. Herbs are also less expensive. However, nearly any substance can cause toxic reactions when used improperly, and plants are no exception. Consult a knowledgeable herbalist or naturopath to help you select the herbs that suit your specific needs.

In this chapter, you can read about the principles behind herbal medicine and how it works. You also have the opportunity to choose herbal remedies for your pain and learn the guidelines for their use. Following the section on remedies, you can learn where to get herbs and how to grow, dry, and store them.

HOW DOES HERBAL MEDICINE WORK?

Plants have active components or "active principles"—organic compounds such as proteins, enzymes, sugars, and vitamins—that work together to treat symptoms with fewer adverse side effects than the isolated active compound. For example, the meadowsweet plant, which contains salicylate compounds like those found in common aspirin, causes less stomach irritation and intestinal bleeding than aspirin taken alone. The other substances in meadowsweet reduce stomach acidity and soothe the stomach lining.

CAN I TREAT MYSELF?

You can treat yourself—with a caveat: we recommend you consult with an herbalist who can help you choose the best herbs to treat your headache pain. Although botanical medicine is not a licensed profession in the United States, there are many trained herbalists you can contact for help in choosing herbal remedies. If you cannot find an herbalist in your area, we recommend you consult with a naturopath, as many of them are trained in botanical medicine. Most people who use herbs are self-taught and consult some of the excellent books that have been written on

TYPES OF HERBAL FORMULAS

Herbal preparations come in several forms. Below are the types we discuss in this chapter, with general basic instructions on how to prepare them. Recipes for specific herbs are included in the section Choosing Herbal Remedies for Your Headache.

- *Infusions* are made from the leaves, flowers, or other soft parts of a plant. They are prepared like teas, use more of the herb than the other forms, and steep longer for greater potency.

  To prepare an infusion, pour 2 cups of boiling water over 2 to 3 tbsp. of the herbs and steep for at least 10 minutes or even overnight in the refrigerator in a tightly covered pot. Strain the liquid. Drink the infusion hot, warm, or cool, depending on the herb and the effect you want. The standard dose for gentle herbs such as peppermint is 1/2–1 cup three to four times a day, more frequently for acute headache.

  Herbal infusions decompose rapidly, so make a fresh batch daily and keep it cool. You can add these preparations to soups, or add honey, lemon, or fruit juices and sweetening for taste.

- *Decoctions* are prepared from the roots, stems, and bark of herbs. To prepare a standard decoction, boil 1 oz. of herb to 1 pint of water in a covered nonmetallic container for 20–30 minutes. Cool and strain the liquid. Doses vary from 1 tsp. to 1 cup taken three to six times a day. Decoctions also deteriorate rapidly and should be made fresh and kept refrigerated for no more than 1 or 2 days.

- *Extracts* are stronger than infusions and are preferred by practitioners because they have a higher concentration of active ingredients. Ready-to-use extracts are available commercially through many health and nutrition stores, pharmacies, herbalists, other natural health practitioners, and by mail order. If you want to make your own, the simplest preparation is a green extract made by thoroughly crushing the juicy parts of the plant and pressing out the juices. For medicinal purposes, 1 oz. of extract equals 1 oz. of the pure, dry herb. Extracts also deteriorate rapidly.

- *Tinctures* are herbal extracts made with alcohol or glycerine instead of water. Because alcohol is a preservative, tinctures have a longer shelf life. Alcohol dissolves the active components of the herbs and keeps them in solution when the remaining plant is sieved. Tinctures are the most potent formulations for most herbal substances. Like extracts (above), they are available commercially.

To prepare a tincture at home, the standard recipe is to steep 2 to 3 tbsp. of herb (dried, fresh, or powdered) in ½ cup of 60-proof vodka (30% alcohol)—enough to keep the plant material wet and covered. Place the herbs and liquid in a tightly sealed glass container (preferably, dark-colored glass to keep out sunlight), label it with the name, date, dosage, and indicated precautions, and keep it out of direct sunlight. Shake or stir the contents at least once per day. If the tincture level goes down, add more spirits to return it to its original level. Two to 6 weeks later, you can strain and squeeze out the plant materials, or just leave them there and pour off the drops as needed. Store the tincture in a cool, shaded or dark place. The usual dose is 10–40 drops in 6–8 oz. of water three to four times a day, although this varies depending on the tincture and the situation.

herbalism and consult herbalists and friends who also use herbs. See the Sources and Suggested Readings for this chapter and Appendix I for information on herb organizations and how to locate herbalists.

CHOOSING HERBAL REMEDIES FOR YOUR HEADACHE

Below is an alphabetical list of some herbs and their indicated uses for headache and headache-related symptoms. Herbal remedies for headache are typically prescribed based on the type of pain—tension or migraine, for example—and the symptoms that may accompany it, such as nausea or fever. Use this section to help you choose an herbal remedy that best matches your pain and symptoms. Most herbs have multiple uses, yet here we describe only those uses as they relate to headache relief.

The following information will help you as you read through the herbal remedy list:

- Under the sections entitled "Part(s) used," *herb* means the entire plant above ground minus tough stems.
- Under "Use(s)," we give you the forms each herbal remedy can take. If you prepare your own remedies, follow the guidelines under each herb or refer to the "Types of Herbal Formulas" box on pp. 188–89. The guidelines are suggestions only.

- Extract dosages are given as a range of drops. Start with the lowest number of drops and increase according to your response.
- Most herbal preparations are gentle and safe. However, as with medicine of any kind, reactions can be highly individual and sometimes extreme. We recommend that you consult an herbalist or other knowledgeable professional for assistance whether you purchase or make your own remedies. If you buy commercially available remedies, follow the package dosage directions.
- All herbs mentioned in this chapter can be purchased in ready-to-use form, as a tea, tincture, extract, or capsules.
- Herbs can be taken either singly or combined with others in a special formula. Commercial brands are available in both forms. Several recipes for making your own combination remedies are also included in this chapter.

Black Cohosh (Cimicifuga racemosa)

Other common names: Black snakeroot, bugwort, bugbane, squawroot, rattleroot, rattlewood, richweed. *Parts used:* Root and rhizome (underground stem). *Uses:* This herb is effective for muscle tension or stress headache, as it directly relaxes muscles and is a sedative for the mind. Black cohosh decreases inflammation and so has some effect, especially with other herbs such as curcumin, on neuralgia. *Tincture:* Prepare the standard recipe and take 10–60 drops in water three times a day. *Decoction:* To prepare, boil ¹/₂ tsp. powdered root per cup of water for 30 minutes. Take 2 tbsp. every few hours, up to 1 cup a day. *Precautions:* If you are taking medications for diabetes or hypertension, check with a knowledgeable pharmacist or health-care practitioner before you take black cohosh. This herb decreases blood pressure and blood sugar levels and can increase the action of medicines you may be taking for diabetes or hypertension. A large dose of the herb may cause nausea, dizziness, dimness of vision, and even headache.

Blessed Thistle (Cnicus benedictus)

Other common names: Saint Benedict thistle, holy thistle, spotted thistle, cardin, bitter thistle. *Parts used:* Root, bark, leaf. *Uses:* This

GUIDELINES FOR USE OF HERBS

Remember these guidelines when you select and use herbs:

- Many people successfully use herbs to treat their headaches themselves. As with any substance, however, misuse may cause adverse effects. It is recommended that you consult an herbal specialist or knowledgeable physician who can guide you in your choices. If you are pregnant, please do not self-treat with herbs without first consulting your physician. Also see Appendix I for helpful organizations and see Sources and Suggested Readings.

- Use glass, porcelain, or enamel heating and cooking containers when preparing remedies; metal can alter the properties of herbs.

- Some herbs interact with other drugs as well as with other herbs. If you are taking conventional drugs, check with a physician, herbalist, or pharmacist who is familiar with the pharmacology of both herbs and prescription agents before you start taking an herbal remedy. Herbal manufacturers and researchers on their staff also may be able to answer your questions over the telephone.

- If fresh herbs are not available, tinctures or freeze-dried herbs contain more of an herb's active ingredients than those dried by traditional methods. Both tinctures and freeze-dried herbs are available commercially.

- When using fresh herbs, you will need to "bruise" the tissues by rubbing them with your hands or against the walls of a nonmetallic container such as glass or porcelain.

- Some people feel nauseated if they take herbs on an empty stomach. To avoid this, take herbs with a meal or snack.

- If you get diarrhea or nausea or experience any problem after taking an herb, stop taking it and call an expert.

herb is most useful for headaches associated with indigestion or fever. *Infusion:* Simmer $1/2$ tsp. in 1 cup water for $1/2$ hour. Drink 1 cup twice daily. If you have a fever, take one of the doses at bedtime; be prepared for sweating to break the fever. *Precaution:* Do not make the infusion any stronger than recommended here, as it may cause vomiting.

Bryony (Bryonia alba)

Common name: Bryony. *Part used:* Herb. *Uses:* Bryony is particularly useful for sharp head pain, head that is tender to touch, headaches that are worse with motion and that go from the front to the back of the head, and pain that may be accompanied by fatigue and excessive perspiration even with small movements. *Tincture:* Prepare the standard recipe and use 1–5 drops in water and take one to three times daily. *Precautions:* Large doses can cause vomiting, diarrhea, congestive headache, cold perspiration, and collapse. Avoid direct contact with the whole fresh plant, as it can cause skin inflammation.

Burdock (Arctium lappa)

Other common names: Clotbur, great bur, cocklebur, lappa. *Parts used:* Roots, leaves, seeds. *Uses:* Burdock is often used as a cleansing herb, as it can promote secretion of bile and stimulate the kidneys to eliminate waste. *Infusion:* Prepare using $1/2$ tsp. of leaves in 8 oz. water. Drink two 8-oz. cups per day. *Extract:* Add 10–25 drops in liquid and drink throughout the day. *Decoction:* Prepare 1 oz. of herb in 24 oz. water. Drink 4 oz. three to four times a day. *Precautions:* The growing plant may cause skin irritation and rash.

Catnip (Nepeta cataria)

Other common names: Catmint, catrup, cat's-wort, field balm. *Parts used:* Leaves and flowers. *Uses:* Catnip is useful for nervous headaches because of its gentle, calming effect. It is also effective against headaches associated with intestinal cramps. *Infusion:* Prepare using 1 tbsp. catnip steeped in 1 cup water and take as needed. *Extract:* Take $1/2$–2 tsp. in 8 oz. warm water and drink 1–2 cups a day. *Precautions:* Do not take if pregnant. Some people experience stomach upset.

Chamomile or Camomile (Anthemis nobilis—*Roman or English Chamomile;* Matricaria chamomilla—*German chamomile*)

Other common names: Roman chamomile, garden chamomile, ground apple. *Part used:* Flowers. *Uses:* Of these two types of chamomile, the English variety is better known for headache relief. Both herbs are mild sedatives and may be helpful for allergy headaches due to an antihistamine component of the herb. For headaches associated with indigestion, heartburn, stomach hyperacidity, stomach cramps, or gas, both herbs have similar healing actions. *Infusion:* Use 2–3 (heaping) tsp. flowers per cup of boiling water. Steep 10–20 minutes and drink as much as needed. *Tincture:* Use $^1/_2$–1 tsp. in water up to three times daily. *Extract:* Use 10–20 drops in water up to three times daily. *Precaution:* Chamomile is generally safe. However, people who are allergic to ragweed should use it with caution.

Devil's Claw (Harpagophytum procumbens)

Common name: Grapple plant. *Parts used:* Root and tuber. *Uses:* Devil's claw is an anti-inflammatory as well as an analgesic that relaxes smooth muscle and lowers blood pressure. Thus, it is effective against headaches caused by muscle, vessel, nerve, and joint inflammation such as temporomandibular joint (TMJ) syndrome, tension headache, neuralgia, and possibly migraine. It is also effective for headache associated with gastrointestinal complaints. *Capsules:* Take up to 1.5 g daily. *Precautions:* Devil's claw should not be used if you are pregnant, and it may cause stomach upset.

Dong Quai (Angelica sylvestris)

Common name: Dong quai. *Part used:* Root. *Uses:* Dong quai is a smooth-muscle relaxant, is somewhat analgesic and relaxing, and is helpful for various headache types. It helps relieve migraine and headaches associated with both high and low blood pressure and fluctuating blood sugar levels. Dong quai is commonly used in Asia to balance hormone levels in women with menstrual and menopausal problems and relieve the headaches these women commonly experience. It is also used to treat allergies to pollen, dust, and other allergens causing upper respiratory symptoms, and so it may offer relief to people with sinusitis due to allergy, especially in combination with other herbs such as nettle. *Infusion:* Prepare using 1 tsp. per cup of water; take 1 tbsp. per dose, up to 2 cups per day. *Precautions:* Do not use if pregnant or if your blood does not clot easily. Do not use dong quai without professional advice if you have estrogen-dependent cancer or a history of cancer. The effect of hormone-influencing herbs on estrogen-dependent tumors varies. On one hand, you may block your own estrogen's stimulation of tumor growth, but on the other hand, you may stimulate the cells with the herb. Benign tumors typically shrink with dong quai.

Ephedra (Ephedra sinica *and Other Species*)

Other common names: Ma huang *(E. sinica),* Mormon tea, desert tea (American species). *Parts used:* Stems and branches. *Uses:* The stems and branches of ephedra contain ephedrine, a nasal decongestant and bronchodilator, which makes this herb effective in treating headache associated with allergies, asthma, and hay fever. The Chinese ephedra contains much more ephedrine than the American species. *Capsules:* Ephedra is available commercially in capsules and as tea; take as directed on the label. *Precautions:* Ephedra can increase blood pressure and should not be taken by those with hypertension, diabetes, heart disease, or thyroid disease. It can be habit forming and can make some people nervous and jittery.

Feverfew (Tanacetum parthenium)

Common name: Headache plant. *Part used:* Herb. *Uses:* Feverfew is effective against migraines, throbbing headaches, and head pain associated with fever, arthritis, or other inflammatory problems. It also can be used to prevent headache, although it may take 2 to 3 months to become effective. Feverfew is also helpful for headache accompanied by nausea (see box on page 195). *Infusion:* Use 2–3 tbsp. per cup of water; take 1–2 cups daily. *Precautions:* Do not use if you are pregnant or if you are allergic to plants of the ragweed family. If you are taking an anticoagulant, avoid feverfew, as it slows clot formation.

Fringe Tree (Chionanthus virginicus)

Other common names: Old man's beard, graybeard tree, poison ash, snowflower, white fringe, snowdrop tree. *Part used:* Bark.

FEVERFEW

Feverfew has been used since ancient times to relieve the discomfort of headache, arthritis, and dizziness. A 1983 study found that 70% of 270 migraine sufferers who took 25 mg freeze-dried pulverized feverfew daily for a prolonged period had decreased frequency and/or intensity of attacks. Another study found that 82 mg feverfew was effective in reducing the number and severity of attacks. These low dosages may be adequate to prevent attacks, although 20 times that amount (1–2 g) may be necessary during an acute attack.

More recent scientific evaluation of feverfew reveals that it has anti-inflammatory and antifever abilities. It also was found to inhibit release of serotonin, another substance identified as a component in migraine.

Uses: Both the dried root bark and the bark can be used to treat migraines and headaches associated with overeating or environmental or food toxicity, which tax the liver enzymes. *Decoction:* Mix 1 tsp. of the bark in 1 cup of boiled water. Take ¹/₃ cup three times a day. *Precautions:* Do not take if pregnant.

Ginger (Zingiber officinale)

Other common names: Black ginger, race ginger. *Part used:* Root. *Use:* Ginger can significantly lessen the severity of migraines, especially those associated with digestive problems. *Infusion:* Mix ¹/₃ tsp. powdered ginger in 1 cup of water and take at the first indication of migraine. As a preventive measure, repeat this infusion four times daily. *Extract:* Take 15 drops in warm water up to three times a day. *Precaution:* Don't swallow powdered ginger without water, as it can burn the esophagus. Ginger is not recommended for, but is often taken by, pregnant women.

Ginseng (Panax sp.)

Common name: American (Panax quinquefolius), Korean ginseng (Panax ginseng), Siberian Ginseng (Eleutherococcus senticosus). *Part used:* Root. *Uses:* Ginseng can relieve tension headaches and migraines, especially those associated with light-headedness, fatigue, post-stress exhaustion, or illness such as flu. It is particularly useful in the elderly and chronically ill, as it improves physical and mental capacity. These two forms of ginseng are generally similar in effect and act as "adaptogens," which balance the body according to the individual's needs. *Infusion:* Use $^1/_2$ tsp. per cup of water, and drink 1–3 cups per day. *Tincture:* Use 5–60 drops in water one to three times a day. *Precautions:* Do not use if you have hay fever, asthma, emphysema, high blood pressure, cardiac arrhythmia, or clotting problems. Ginseng is expensive and is often "cut" with other substances. Get a reliable brand.

Guarana (Paulina cupana)

Common name: Guarana. *Part used:* Seeds. *Uses:* The seeds of this South American plant contain up to 5% caffeine—more than in coffee beans. As is coffee, an infusion of guarana is effective against migraine and mild depression. *Infusion:* Prepare using 1 tsp. per cup of water and drink 1–2 cups per day. *Capsules:* Take as directed on package. Guarana is usually combined with other herbs. *Precaution:* Do not take guarana if pregnant. This herb is as addictive as coffee and causes many of the same side effects.

Hops (Humulus lupulus)

Common name: Hops. *Part used:* Flowers. *Uses:* Hops are good for nervous headaches and headaches accompanied by nausea or insomnia. *Infusion.* Use 1–2 tsp. per cup of water and steep for 5 minutes. Drink 1 cup before bedtime or 1–2 cups per day as needed for nervous headache. *Precautions:* Hops should not be taken by pregnant women or women with estrogen-dependent breast cancer.

Lavender (Lavandula officinalis)

Other common names: Garden lavender, spike lavender, common lavender. *Part used:* Flowers. *Uses:* Lavender alone is good for nervous headaches, or it can be combined with an equal amount of lady's slipper or valerian. (See Aromatherapy in this chapter to learn how to use lavender oil for headache.) *Infusion.* Prepare using 1 tsp. per cup of water and take as needed. *Precaution:* No known side effects.

Milk Thistle (Silybum marianum)

Other common name: St. Mary's thistle. *Parts used:* Seeds, stems. *Uses:* Milk thistle is effective for headaches associated with food toxins, such as monosodium glutamate (MSG), nitrites, and caffeine. It contains a compound called sylmarin (or silymarin), which helps the liver to regenerate and detoxify many potentially harmful toxins in the body. *Capsules:* This is the most effective form. Take according to package directions. *Tincture or extract:* Take 10–40 drops in water up to three times a day. *Food:* Mix 1 tbsp. powdered milk thistle seeds with food; this can be taken two to three times a day. *Precaution:* Milk thistle can have a mild laxative effect.

Oat (Avena sativa)

Common name: Oat. *Parts used:* Seeds, straw. *Uses:* This herb is ideal for headaches from nervous exhaustion or depression when some, but not a lot, of sedation is needed. Oats are also useful for headache associated with nicotine or other stimulant withdrawal. *Infusion:* Add 1–2 tsp. dried straw per cup of water and drink as needed. *Tincture or extract:* Made from the seeds; take 10–20 drops in water up to three times a day. *Precaution:* No known side effects.

Passionflower (Passiflora incarnata)

Common name: Passionflower. *Parts used:* Flowers and vine. *Uses:* Passionflower contains sedating substances and is good for nervous headaches and insomnia. (Also see "Combination Remedies" box on page 199. It also relieves muscle spasm. *Infusion:* Standard; take as needed. *Tincture:* Use 10–30 drops in water as needed. *Precautions:* This herb can bring on menstruation; avoid in pregnancy.

Peppermint (Mentha piperita)

Other common names: Brandy mint, balm mint, curled mint, lamb mint. *Part used:* Leaves. *Uses:* Peppermint can relieve headaches when taken internally, and the odor of peppermint, when applied externally, also can trigger relief. It is particularly effective for headaches accompanied by nausea and gas. (Also see Aromatherapy in this chapter.) *Infusion:* Prepare a standard infusion and drink 2–3 cups, as needed. *Extract:* Add 5–15 drops to water and take up to three times daily. *Precaution:* Do not use peppermint if you have a hiatal hernia, as this herb relaxes the lower esophageal sphincter and can let stomach acid rise. Spearmint and other mints do not have these medicinal qualities.

Scullcap (Scutellaria lateriflora)

Other common names: Skullcap, blue skullcap, blue pimpernel, hoodwart, hooded willow herb, mad weed, helmet flower. *Part used:* Leaves. *Uses:* This herb is prescribed for tension headaches, especially those associated with mental or physical exhaustion. Scullcap also quiets the nervous system and reduces insomnia. *Infusion:* Prepare a standard infusion and let stand about 15 minutes. Then strain and take 2–3 oz. every few hours. *Capsules:* Take one up to three times daily. *Extract:* Take 3–12 drops in water once daily. *Precaution:* Large amounts of the extract can cause giddiness, confusion, and twitching.

Tetterwort (Chelidonium majus)

Common name: Celandine. *Part used:* Herb. *Uses:* Tetterwort treats headache from overindulgence of food, alcohol, or drugs and from environmental toxicity, which taxes the liver. *Infusion:* Use $1/2$ oz. dried fresh herb in 2 cups boiling water. *Tincture or extract:* Add 5–10 drops to water as a single preparation and divide into three equal doses taken daily. *Precautions:* High doses can cause nausea, liver pain, tenderness, chest pain, coughing, and breathing difficulties.

Valerian (Valeriana officinalis)

Other common names: English valerian, German valerian, great wild valerian, Vermont valerian, vandal root, all-heal. *Part used:* Root. *Uses:* This herb treats headache associated with anxiety and nervous tension. *Infusion:* Use $1/2$–1 tsp. powdered root per cup of water and take before bed. *Capsules:* Take one up to three times daily. *Tincture:* Take 1–2 tsp. in a glass of water daily. To increase valerian's effectiveness, take it with hops for headache caused by acute stress and insomnia. *Extract:* Mix 10–30 drops in liquid as a single preparation and divide into three equal doses taken daily. *Precautions:* Start with small amounts. Do not exceed the recommended dose and do not boil the root. Poisoning may result if you take very large amounts for more than 2 weeks, but it is very safe in standard doses. If you are under stress, take valerian in small amounts only until you see your reaction. Valerian can cause a hangover feeling and, rarely, can cause increased anxiety. However, it is the single most effective herbal sedative commonly available.

White Willow (Salix alba)

Other common names: White willow, salacin willow, willow bark, withe, withy. *Parts used:* Leaves, bark. *Uses:* White willow is used to treat tension headaches, migraines, and head pain associated with any type of inflammation, including fever, arthritis pain, and menstrual cramps. This herb contains salacin, which metabolizes to acetylsalicylic acid, or "aspirin," which is the source of its pain-relieving powers. *Decoction:* Boil 1 tsp. bark in 3 cups water for 1/2 hour. Take 1 tbsp. every 4–6 hours to a maximum of 1 cup per day. *Precautions:* Take white willow only as directed; like aspirin, it can cause stomach distress, although reportedly less so. Do not use white willow if you have gastritis or ulcers.

COMBINATION REMEDIES

Combination herbal remedies are available in commercial formulations, usually in infusion (tea) or capsule form. If you want to make your own, here are a few recipes.

- For headache accompanied by nausea or nervousness, prepare a standard infusion using equal parts of chamomile, peppermint, and catnip to total 2–3 tbsp. herbs in 2 cups of water. Drink 1–2 cups, or as needed.

- For headaches caused by nervousness and accompanied by insomnia, prepare a standard infusion using equal parts of passionflower, valerian, hops, and catnip or scullcap to total 2–3 tbsp. herbs in 2 cups of water. Drink as needed and before bed.

WHERE TO GET HERBS

As herbal medicine grows in popularity, more and more health- and natural-food stores, holistic pharmacies, natural medicine practitioners, and mail-order companies offer ready-made herbal remedies as infusions, capsules, tinctures, and extracts. If you prefer to prepare your own remedies, dried herbs, either prepacked or in bulk, are available commercially through the same outlets. A list of commercial herb growers and suppliers of herbal remedies appears in Appendix II. Some people, however, enjoy having an herb garden in their back yard or on their windowsills. If you want to grow your own, here are some tips.

Growing Your Own

A few pots on your porch or a small plot in your vegetable garden is all you'll need to supply you with headache remedies. Contact your local nurseries and greenhouses for seeds or starter plants. Owing to rising interest in herbalism, many of these businesses now carry a varied assortment of herbs. You also can order from any of the commercial herb growers in the United States (see Appendix II). Organic varieties are also available.

Drying and Storing Herbs

To prepare most herbal formulas, you need to start with dried materials. Two common drying methods are traditional (tie the herbs in bunches and hang them in a warm, dry, dark area until they crumble) and oven or solar oven drying (a faster approach involving placing the herbs on a cookie sheet or screen in a 95-degree oven or using a produce dryer). The faster herbs are dried, the more the aromatic volatile oils are retained.

Once the herbs are dry, you can strip the leaves to store them as is or make a powder using a mortar and pestle, grinder, or blender. To retain herbs' medicinal potency and flavor, store them in ceramic or opaque glass containers with tight-fitting lids to prevent moisture and pests from finding their way into the jars. Use dark glass, as light can destroy herbal potency. Keep the amount of oxygen in the containers to a minimum by keeping them as full as possible. As you use the herbs, fill up the empty space with cotton. Most properly stored herbs are potent for at least 1 year. Bark and roots last longer when stored whole.

Herbal medicine has been used for millennia to treat conditions such as headache. The herbal remedies presented in this chapter have withstood the test of time because they have offered relief to people around the world. We hope you will find them effective as a part of your herbal medicine cabinet.

AROMATHERAPY

Aromatherapy is a form of herbalism in which the fragrance of the plant's essential oils is used for its healing effects. Essential oils are the potent, aromatic substances that are formed in minute glands in leaves, roots, wood, flowers, or fruit of a plant. These oils are typically pressed out of the plant and saved in their concentrated form and are then inhaled from the container directly, added to a bath and inhaled while bathing, or applied to the skin of the face or neck with massage or compresses.

The primary effect of essential oils is olfactory (sense of smell); however, oils are absorbed well through the skin. Many have local and systemic anti-inflammatory action on joints and soft tissues and also moisturize and protect the skin. Some plant substances, when applied, accelerate the healing process and decrease pain locally. Essential oils are popular for use during self-massage of the face and neck and self-treatment for skin and local problems.

HOW DOES AROMATHERAPY WORK?

Each essential oil can contain hundreds of different, sometimes complex chemicals that have coevolved for the benefit of the plant and to attract pollinating birds and insects.

Essential oils enter the body through the nose or through the skin. When the vapors are inhaled, they may directly affect emotional processes, as the areas of the brain that process smell are closely associated with the areas that control the emotions and the autonomic physical functions. It is not completely known how aromatherapy can relieve symptoms such as headache, but aromatherapists believe that when the chemical components of the essential oils reach the brain, they impact on physical symptoms and our perception of those symptoms.

When the oils are absorbed through the skin, they reach the blood stream and lymph system in about 20 minutes, depending on the thickness of skin and amount of fat and blood supply where applied. From the blood stream, the oils reach organs and systems throughout the body.

WHAT DOES AN AROMATHERAPIST DO?

An aromatherapist is likely to gather information about your symptoms, medical history, and especially your emotional state. Unless the therapist is also a physician, however, she or he is not licensed to diagnose and treat. The therapist can share the art of aromatherapy with you as an educational experience, and you can experiment and learn by experience what works for you.

Once the therapist has prepared a blend that she or he believes best fits your symptoms, you will be asked to smell it. It is essential that you like the smell. If your aromatherapist is licensed to do massage, she or he may apply the oils for you. If not, you will receive recommendations and instructions on how to use them at home. Many aromatherapists, however, practice other natural therapies, such as reflexology or massage, and the combination approach is often most effective.

AROMATHERAPY REMEDIES FOR HEADACHES

Very little research has been done on the therapeutic effectiveness of aromatherapy. According to the International Federation of Aromatherapists, it "enhances well-being, relieves stress, and helps in the rejuvenation and regeneration of the human body" and can help with migraines, sleeping problems, moderate depression, digestive disorders, and other conditions. Several studies conducted by nurses have shown it to be useful in reducing tension and treating sinusitis and menstrual problems, among other disorders.

Below are some essential oils that aromatherapists recommend most often for various types of headache pain. The list carries explanations of which oils combine well and how to use them. The only "rules" to combining essential oils are as follows: (1) prepare a combination of oils that smells good to you, (2) select those that combine well, and (3) do not mix more than five different oils together, as this decreases their synergistic abilities (see "Carrier Oils" box below for instructions on how to mix oils). If you have migraine and are sensitive to touch, inhalation of the oils rather than massage is suggested.

You can get essential oils at health-food or herb stores, at homeopathic pharmacies, from aromatherapists, or by mail order (see Appendix II).

- **Basil** *(Ocimum basilicum):* Blends well with lavender. Use for tension and migraine headaches accompanied by nausea and vomiting.
- **Eucalyptus** *(Eucalyptus globulus):* Has analgesic properties and is often used in a headache blend, especially for pain accompanied by fever. Tends to dominate in a mixture and can be irritative, so use sparingly.
- **Lavender** *(Lavandula officinalis):* Blends well with many other oils. Used for migraines, tension headaches, and headaches associated with colds and flu. Known for its ability to balance and soothe.

CARRIER OILS

Undiluted essential oils are potent and can cause skin reactions, so they need to be mixed with a carrier oil or lotion before use. Cold-pressed jojoba oil is one of the best and suits all skin types; cold-pressed vegetable oils such as safflower, sesame, and sweet almond also are recommended. If you have dry skin, use wheat-germ, olive, or avocado oils, which are heavier and seal in moisture more completely. Taking a bath or shower before applying the oils increases skin moisture. Carrier lotions are another option. These are made from emulsified oil and water, which makes them non-greasy and easy to apply.

The basic diluting instructions are as follows: add 5 drops (total) of the oils you have chosen to ½ fluid oz. carrier oil or lotion; add 10 drops to 1 fluid oz.; add 20 drops to 2 fluid oz. Store any unused portions in a dark-glass dropper bottle that has a tight screw-top. Dropper bottles are easy to use.

- **Lemon balm** *(Melissa officinalis):* This oil is included in blends used to treat migraines. It may cause skin irritation in some people.
- **Peppermint** *(Mentha piperita):* Use this strong oil sparingly, as it can irritate the skin. Peppermint blends well with rosemary and is used for migraines and tension headaches and for headaches that accompany colds or flu.
- **Roman chamomile** *(Anthemis nobilis):* A dominant herb that mixes well with lavender. Used for headaches accompanied by depression, nervousness, irritability, stomach upset, restlessness, and insomnia.
- **Rose** *(Rosa damascena):* Used in treatment of migraines—mix equal parts of rose and balm in carrier oil (see box on page 203). Effective for menstrual problems, depression, and sorrow.
- **Rosemary** *(Rosmarinus officinalis):* Used for migraines. Is a stimulant and complements lavender well.
- **Sweet marjoram** *(Origanum majorana):* Used for migraines and headaches associated with stress, anxiety, grief, or other negative emotions. Blends well with rosemary, lavender, and eucalyptus.

GENERAL USES FOR ESSENTIAL OILS

Following are some ways to use essential oils:

- Inhalation is most effective if done soon after symptoms appear. As a general treatment for tension headaches and headaches associated with sinus congestion or menstruation, sprinkle 2 drops each of undiluted lavender, peppermint, and sweet marjoram on a tissue. First, inhale gently; if the smell is pleasant to you, then inhale deeply three times. For migraine, add 1 drop of lemon balm to these three oils.
- When using oils for massage, apply diluted oils over pressure points, especially your temples, behind your ears, in the hollows on the outside corners of your eye bone, and in the nape of your neck.
- When using oils in a bath, add a few drops to warm—not hot—bath water. Because oils do not dissolve, swish the water around periodically. If you have dry skin, dilute the

essential oils in 2 tsp. carrier oil before you add them to the bath. Relax in the bath for 10–20 minutes and gently breathe in the vapors.

CHOOSING, PREPARING, AND USING ESSENTIAL OILS

If you try aromatherapy yourself, remember these guidelines:

- Keep essential oils away from children and away from your eyes. If you do get oil into your eye, flush it out immediately with lots of water. If you have sweet almond oil on hand, a few drops in the irritated eye can dilute the offending oil.
- Never take essential oils internally or apply to broken or irritated skin or pimples without the guidance of an aromatherapist or physician.
- Do not apply undiluted essential oils to your skin unless specifically instructed to do so.
- When you test the smell of essential oils, sniff gently: the effects can be potent. Allow a few minutes to pass between tests so you can "digest" your response to each oil or blend.
- Test a drop of oil on your skin before using it liberally. Place 1 drop of carrier oil or lotion (see box on page 203) on your arm where you can see it, and wait for 12 hours. If you do not have an adverse reaction, dilute 1 drop essential oil in 1/2 tsp. carrier oil or lotion and rub this combination on your other arm. If no reaction occurs after 12 hours, you can probably use the combination oil without a reaction. Reactions can occur at any time to any substance taken orally, topically, or through inhalation.

Aromatherapy is gaining attention as a reliever of stress and headache pain by aromatherapists and nursing professionals, especially in the United States, Great Britain, and France. It is an easy technique to use either alone or as a complement to self-massage or application of compresses during progressive relaxation, meditation, or guided imagery.

The use of plants and their essential oils in medicine and healing has a long history, as far back as 3000 B.C. Both herbal medicine and aromatherapy derive their power from the plant kingdom, a resource about which we are becoming more knowledgeable and one that is the subject of increasing research. Thus, the next time you prepare an infusion, mix up a tincture, or combine essential oils for your headache pain, know that you are part of a long healing tradition and an evolving one.

13

HOMEOPATHY

In the United States, the medical community is now slowly warming to homeopathy as a legitimate medical therapy. Homeopathy is a natural medicine approach based on the concept that symptoms, such as headache, are the body's way of trying to heal itself and therefore should not be suppressed. In this approach, homeopaths treat a disease or illness with a very minute amount of a substance that, if taken in larger doses, would cause the same symptoms they are treating in people without symptoms. Thus, homeopathic remedies, which are derived from plants, minerals, or animals and occasionally from a person's own fluids, stimulate the body to heal itself.

This idea is not totally foreign to physicians who are familiar with the body's response to very small amounts of substances. Immunizations, for example, are actually minute doses of inactive whole or parts of bacteria or viruses administered to stimulate the body to produce the antibodies necessary to fight specific diseases. The result is increased levels of antibodies. For allergies, your physician may give you a dilution of the allergen, the same substance that is causing your allergic reactions, and the immune reaction decreases. In both cases, the minute dose brings the body toward a normal balance.

The growing interest in homeopathy by the general public is also bringing homeopathy into the mainstream. *Time* magazine, for example, published an article in which the U.S. Food and Drug Administration reported that in recent years, the sale of homeopathic remedies has increased by 1,000 percent and is still growing. Studies showing the effectiveness of homeopathy are being published in mainstream medical journals.

In Great Britain, more than 40 percent of physicians commonly refer patients to homeopathic physicians, while about 30 percent of families in France and 20 percent in Germany use homeopathic remedies. More than 100,000 practitioners prescribe homeopathic remedies in India.

In this chapter, we talk about how homeopathic remedies are used to treat headaches and other symptoms that accompany head pain. You will learn how remedies are prescribed, discover the role of a homeopath, and have the opportunity to choose a remedy for your head pain.

HOW DO HOMEOPATHIC REMEDIES WORK?

Homeopathic remedies stimulate your body's natural defenses and allow them to do what they do naturally: heal and return your system to its natural state of homeostasis, or balance. Homeopathy views symptoms as signals from the body that something is out of balance, and each remedy is given to provoke the entire being into balance again. If, for example, your head feels as if there is a band wrapped around it, you are shaking, and you feel very tired, you might try gelsemium. Why?

Homeopathy is based on the "law of similars" or "let likes be cured by likes." This means that while a relatively large amount of a substance given to a healthy person will produce certain symptoms, a greatly diluted amount of the same substance will cure the same symptoms. If you were to munch on a gelsemium root, you would develop all of the symptoms just described, yet a minute homeopathic dose of the same root, like that in a gelsemium tablet, can cure these symptoms. This medical approach takes its name from the combining forms *homeo-* ("like") and *-pathy* ("disease"). It differs from the way conventional (or *allopathic*, meaning "different disease") medicine is practiced. In homeopathy, symptoms such as headache and fever, for example, are seen as the body's attempts to heal itself, and so the remedy you or the homeopath choose would allow these symptoms to run their course and let healing occur. In allopathic medicine, symptoms are viewed as something to suppress and mask with medication, which may provide relief but does not address the underlying cause of the pain.

Homeopathic remedies go to the core of the pain, and they do this in a seemingly contradictory way: the more a remedy goes through dilution and succussion, the greater is its potency, even if no molecules of the substance are present in the final dilution. A 1M formulation, for example, has been through potentization (see How Homeopathic Remedies Are Made, below) 1,000 times and has a very high potency. Why does this process of potentization result in a more potent remedy? According to quantum physics, all physical substances are composed of energy and leave behind an energy field, like footsteps in the sand, as they move or change position. When a homeopathic remedy goes through repeated potentization, no molecules of the original substance may be present in the resulting remedy. However, "footsteps" of the molecules *are* in these remedies and exist at high energy—and hence, high potency—levels. Thus, homeopathy is often classified as "bioenergy medicine" or simply "energy medicine" because similar to acupuncture and therapeutic touch, it effects the life force directly.

HOW HOMEOPATHIC REMEDIES ARE MADE

Homeopathic remedies are derived from a mother tincture that is prepared, like an herbal tincture, by mixing the chosen plant part, mineral, or animal substance with a solvent, usually alcohol. One drop of this tincture is mixed with 99 drops of water or alcohol. This mixture is shaken well (the process is called succussion), and the resulting formulation is called 1C. When one drop of the 1C formulation is added to 99 drops of water or alcohol and shaken, the result is a 2C mixture. This dilution and shaking procedure is known as potentization and is repeated again and again, sometimes hundreds of times (see "Homeopathic Potencies" box on page 210).

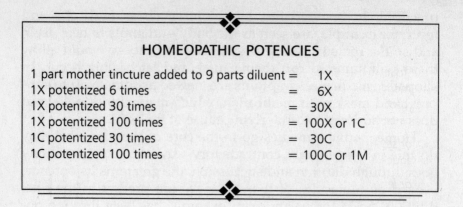

HOMEOPATHIC POTENCIES

1 part mother tincture added to 9 parts diluent =	1X
1X potentized 6 times =	6X
1X potentized 30 times =	30X
1X potentized 100 times =	100X or 1C
1C potentized 30 times =	30C
1C potentized 100 times =	100C or 1M

Many commercial homeopathics are available in a dose of 6X, which is a very safe starting dose. For acute headache, a 30C dose taken three times a day is common. Individuals with chronic headache may require more potent doses, such as 1M or 10M, which should be taken under the guidance of an experienced homeopath (see "constitutional remedy" under Your First Visit to a Homeopath, in this chapter). See the box on page 211 for general dosing guidelines.

UNDERSTANDING HOMEOPATHIC DOSAGES

For treatment of headaches and migraines, dosing is usually as drops or tablets (sugar pills), which have been infused with the remedy and have either a sweet taste or no taste at all. Both of these forms make them especially simple to give to children. When you follow the directions of your physician or those on the label of commercial brands, they are a safe, effective alternative to conventional medical treatments.

Dosage intervals as well as the dosages themselves are highly variable and depend on the individual homeopath and the manufacturer of the remedy. If a small dose only partially corrects your symptoms, you might need a higher potency or an additional homeopathic remedy. If symptoms change, you will likely need another remedy. Some changes and effects can be expected and are managed best by an experienced homeopath.

DOSING GUIDELINES

The following dosing schedules are a general guideline. You can make adjustments as needed or as your homeopath prescribes. If using a commercial product, follow the package directions. One dose usually equals 2–3 drops or pills.

- *For severe, acute pain:* Take one dose every 15 minutes for 1 hour, then reduce the dose to one tablet or pill every 30 minutes until you get relief.

- *For less urgent conditions:* Take one dose three times daily and note any changes in your pain and other symptoms you may have.

- *Persistent condition:* Same as for less urgent conditions. If, however, the headache continues or increases in intensity, see your medical professional.

If your symptoms get worse after taking a remedy, that may indicate that the remedy will be effective for ultimate cure. This temporary increase in pain, known as a "proving," is so named because it "proves" that a particular remedy is working. Not everyone has this reaction, however. Some homeopaths believe proving is necessary for an effective cure and prescribe more potent remedies to induce one. Others prefer to dispense lower-potency remedies and usually avoid the proving process.

If you start to feel an improvement but then it "stalls" or reaches a plateau, restart the remedy at a higher potency or see a homeopath for a new remedy. In a rare case in which worsening symptoms are accompanied by fever, confusion, or other new conditions, contact your homeopath or physician immediately.

SINGLE DOSING

Most homeopaths follow a single-remedy approach in which the patient takes only one remedy at a time. If one does not bring relief, it is stopped and another one is tried. Therefore, a person with headache accompanied by nausea and cough would take a single homeopathic remedy that best matched all the symptoms.

In homeopathy, if other symptoms replace the primary ones because of a remedy, it is said that the homeopath has approached another layer. Thus, the homeopath will change the remedy to balance this "new person," complete with newly emerged symptoms, and move to deeper layers of healing. Meanwhile, the individual "blossoms" emotionally as well as symptomatically: unrelated problems resolve, energy levels change, social involvement, optimism, and personal relationships flourish. The one remedy prescribed for the "old" person evolves to new remedies as the individual evolves. Homeopaths do not give remedies to counter the effects of other ones. This treatment approach leads some people to say, "Homeopathy treats people; conventional medicine treats symptoms."

COMBINATION DOSING

Although traditional homeopaths follow the single-dosing concept, some practitioners combine remedies. Combination remedies are also available commercially in many health-food stores and pharmacies. If you purchase commercial products, follow package directions. Consult with a practitioner who is knowledgeable about combination dosing before you attempt to prepare your own combination remedies; however, commercial combinations are very effective.

CAN I TREAT MY HEADACHE MYSELF?

Many individuals successfully treat their own headache pain using homeopathic remedies. Of the more than 2,000 homeopathic remedies available, 100 to 200 are used most often. These remedies are becoming increasingly more available for people who want to self-treat. For most headache pain, homeopathic remedies often work much more dramatically and rapidly than most traditional drugs, and they also are less expensive.

Your unique physical and emotional symptoms and general sensitivities all need to be considered when choosing the most appropriate homeopathic remedy for your headache pain, and homeopaths are specially trained in this kind of diagnostic technique. They also know when to alter your prescription based on how you react to a given remedy. It is recommended, therefore, that you consult a professional homeopath for guidance when choosing a remedy, especially if your headache is chronic or associated with an underlying medical condition such as inflammation or infection. Chronic headaches typically are not permanently cured by intensive, short-term use of homeopathic remedies. In such cases, it is strongly recommended you work closely with an experienced, intuitive therapeutic specialist who can prescribe a constitutional remedy (see Your First Visit to a Homeopath, below).

Homeopathy is the fastest growing form of medicine in the world, and with its increased popularity has come a growing influx of prepared, over-the-counter homeopathic remedies available from practitioners, corner drugstores, or health-food stores. These remedies are prepared by homeopathic pharmacies that follow the guidelines of the *Homeopathic Pharmacopoeia of the United States*, the official manufacturing manual recognized by the U.S. Food and Drug Administration. (For a list of homeopathic remedy suppliers, see Appendix II.)

YOUR FIRST VISIT TO A HOMEOPATH

The first time you visit a homeopath, you will probably be pleasantly surprised. One woman describes it as being like talking with a new friend. Rather than the average of 7 minutes that conventional physicians spend with each patient, homeopaths spend an hour or more with their patients. Homeopaths believe it is essential to have a complete picture of an individual's state of health—physical, emotional, spiritual—and habits and thoughts in order to make an accurate diagnosis and choose the best remedy to return the body to health and balance. A good homeopath listens and observes your speech, manners, posture, and even how you dress: all are considered along with your symptoms and your medical and family history.

You will be asked questions about yourself, your job, and family, and what you like to do. Some questions may seem a little odd; for example, did you talk in your sleep as a child? Are your hands and feet hot or cold at night? All your answers are important, because they help the homeopath put together a "constitutional profile," which helps him or her determine the remedy that will cure you. This is the approach you can use, in a simplified form, to select your own homeopathic remedy in the section Selecting a Homeopathic Remedy by Your Symptoms. This method was developed in the 1790s by Samuel Hahnemann, the father of modern homeopathy, and his colleagues. They conducted experiments with homeopathic remedies and observed that different types of people reacted strongly to certain substances. They categorized these individuals and noted similarities among them, including body type, appearance, personality, and diseases they had. People who respond well to belladonna, for example, tend to have a sturdy build, vigorous mental and physical energy, and be in apparent robust health.

If you go to your homeopath for chronic headache, she or he will develop a constitutional profile of you to determine which "constitutional remedy" will best relieve your pain. Constitutional remedies are said to work deeper than acute remedies to treat more persistent conditions such as chronic headache. Constitutional remedies may be taken once and repeated in high doses over several months, and they can be prescribed for daily use. Every person is unique and has different needs; therefore, prescribing of homeopathic remedies is extremely variable, as is the amount of time it takes to heal whatever condition is causing the pain. They strengthen your bioenergy force and gradually reduce the number and severity of each episode of head pain. These remedies need to be prescribed and monitored by an experienced homeopath.

If your homeopathic physician suspects an underlying condition, he or she may ask you to undergo additional medical tests or refer you to a specialist (see Chapter 2). Homeopathy works very well with many standard medical therapies; however, always consult with your physician and your homeopath before starting any type of drug or homeopathic remedy program.

GUIDELINES FOR USING HOMEOPATHIC REMEDIES

Here are some general guidelines to remember when you use and store your homeopathic remedies:

- Keep remedies in the containers in which they were supplied or transfer them to airtight glass containers without contaminating them with strong odors or by touching the skin or unclean surfaces.
- Store remedies away from strong light, intense heat, or any substance that has a strong odor, such as perfumes, moth balls, or menthol.
- Take the remedy on a "clean tongue." Make sure your mouth is free from food, beverages, mouthwash or toothpaste, candies, or tobacco smoke for about 30 minutes before taking a dose.
- Avoid using other conventional medicine, such as aspirin, laxatives, or nasal drops, while using a homeopathic remedy. If you are taking prescription medications, consult with a physician knowledgeable about the effects of both types of remedies.
- Homeopathic remedies can be applied or swallowed; however, they are usually taken as a liquid or a pellet dissolved under the tongue so absorption can occur through the mucous membranes of the mouth. This eliminates the need to take them with water.

SELECTING A HOMEOPATHIC REMEDY BY YOUR SYMPTOMS

We have selected a handful of the most common and effective homeopathic remedies for headache. Browse through the following choices, listed by primary general symptoms in boldface italics. Find the symptoms that best describe your headache pain. These primary symptoms are key; however, the remedy is more likely to work if the description fits you and the pain in more ways than not, so also see which of the symptoms in regular type also match yours. Not all of the characteristics will describe you exactly; simply find the remedy that is closest to your symptoms. And although some of the symptoms and remedies may sound odd, they have proven effective over the years and continue to be used by tens of thousands of people around the world.

Homeopaths use this same approach: choosing a remedy by matching the symptoms with the pattern of symptoms that a specific remedy produces. For example, two women may suffer from premenstrual headache, both reporting sharp pain, like a nail is being hammered into their head. One may be very sensitive to light and noise during her attack and finds some relief by staying in a dark, quiet room and sleeping. The other's head feels heavy, as if it is congested, and also experiences a build-up of nausea and feels much better after she vomits.

Although both women have headache that is triggered by the same situation and even have the same kind of headache pain, their symptom patterns are not the same. Therefore, a homeopath might prescribe sepia for the first woman and ignatia for the second; substances that, in large quantities, produce the symptoms these women experience along with their headache.

For dosing instructions on the remedies listed below, follow the package directions or the advice of your health-care practitioner or homeopathic pharmacist; also see Understanding Homeopathic Dosages in this chapter. You may have to try several remedies before you find one that works for you.

- *Headache brought on by any type of **injury** to any part of the body, especially right after the injury, and if you are stunned or confused; also **hot head with cold body** and dry mouth.* Damp and cold conditions and walking make pain worse; staying dry and changing position often alleviate the pain. *Remedy: arnica.*

  Arnica is from *Arnica montana,* or leopard's bane. The remedy is made from the whole fresh plant, just the root, or from the dried flowers. It is most helpful after trauma for sore, bruised emotions and especially for people who refuse to admit they are in trouble and will not see a doctor.

- *Violent **throbbing pain with sudden onset**.* Symptoms include extreme sensitivity to light, noise, even the lightest touch, smell, and motion, which cause new waves of pain. Other common symptoms include dizziness that causes falling to the side or backward, high fever with flushed face, and cold hands and feet. Pain is typically worse in the forehead and may extend to the back of the head. The pain is better when sitting and worse when lying down, climbing stairs, and moving down a slope or stairway. Firm pressure applied to the head offers some relief. *Remedy: belladonna.* If this is the appropriate remedy, relief will be rapid.

Belladonna *(Atropa belladonna)* is the most common remedy for headache with fever that is usually accompanied by sore throat with swollen glands. The entire fresh plant is used to make the homeopathic remedy. It works best in children and in individuals who are generally in excellent health and have a sturdy build.

- *Splitting, crushing headache* **aggravated by motion,** *even slight motion of the eyes or head.* Firm pressure alleviates pain, but slight touch makes it worse. Symptoms include a steady ache, perhaps with a feeling of heaviness or fullness. The pain typically occurs in the forehead and over the left eye. Nausea, constipation, vomiting, and fainting may occur; irritability, physical weakness, a desire to be left alone (this latter symptom is true of most headaches except those helped by pulsatilla), and dry lips, throat, tongue, and mouth are common. Relief comes from staying in cool rooms and open air, lying perfectly still, and lying on the painful side. Warm rooms, sunlight, eating, exertion, and motion make it worse. *Remedy: bryonia.*

Bryonia *(Bryonia alba)* remedies are made from the entire fresh plant. The plant's therapeutic effect on fibrous tissues, nerve coating, and other areas that become inflamed also make it effective in individuals with rheumatism. Bryonia is most effective in people who are above average weight, have dark hair and a dark complexion, and are irritated or angered easily.

- **Daily,** *intermittent fever with* **debilitating sweats** *and great anxiety; strong throbbing of neck arteries, and* **head feels like it will burst.** Head pain is typically one sided; scalp is hypersensitive to touch, so that even combing the hair is painful. The pain is aggravated by bright lights and open-air spaces. *Remedy: china.*

China is derived from the dried bark of a South American evergreen shrub *(Cinchona calisaya),* which contains quinine. Artistic individuals usually respond well to china.

This remedy is generally reserved for very ill individuals who have great head pain.

- *Bursting headache caused by **eyestrain** from reading fine print or long hours in front of a computer screen or associated with a cold.* The eyes are red, hot, or dazed. Cold and dampness make the pain worse; movement and walking in open spaces alleviates the pain. *Remedy: euphrasia.*

  Euphrasia is made from the entire fresh *Euphrasia officinalis* plant, also known as eyebright. This homeopathic remedy was traditionally used for eye ailments.

- ***Eyeballs painful;** person feels **listless, apathetic,** and has dull, frontal head pain.* Head pain is worse with bending forward. *Remedy: fringe tree.*

  Fringe tree (*Chionanthus virginicus*) is useful for many types of headache pain. When taken for several weeks, it can break a cycle of sick headaches.

- ***Quivering and shaking; pain resembles a band wrapped around the head** and begins at the back of the head; or there is neck pain that extends to the rest of the head or to the forehead.* Headache pain comes on gradually and is often accompanied by listlessness and fatigue as well as visual disturbances, such as dimness of vision, dilated pupils, and heavy eyelids. The pain is worse in the morning; noise, light, lying down, and motion aggravate the pain; urination, perspiration, and taking a nap with the head raised on a pillow alleviate it. *Remedy: gelsemium.*

  Gelsemium remedies come from the root of the fresh *Gelsemium sempervirens*, yellow jasmine. Individuals who feel weak or have low stamina, weak kidneys or bladder, or joint pains respond well to gelsemium.

- ***Throbbing** in any part of the head **in synch with full, bounding pulse.*** Head pain is worse with heat, motion, or when the head is laid on a pillow with the neck bent; pain is alleviated by being in open-air spaces. *Remedy: glonoinum.*

  Glonoinum's source is liquid nitroglycerin. Women with high blood pressure, especially those who are overweight, respond well to this remedy. Glonoinum is good for congestive headache caused by excess heat or cold, and for when the head feels heavy and head pain is accompanied by confusion.

- *Head feels heavy and congested; headaches with **strong emotion or fainting.*** The head feels hollow. Headache is caused by anger, grief, and loss; emotions are predominant and interfere with daily life. Facial muscle twitches may occur. Pain often ends after vomiting and excess urination. The pain is worse with stooping, coffee, and smelling tobacco smoke. *Remedy: ignatia.*

  Ignatia *(Ignatia amara,* or St. Ignatius's bean) remedies are made from the seed pods of this plant, which contain strychnine. In homeopathic doses, the amount of strychnine is so minute that it does not cause problems. Individuals who respond best to ignatia tend to be emotionally sensitive and unpredictable; artistic women usually have good response.

- *Bursting or throbbing pain with **loss of vision or visual disturbances.*** Head pain may occur as congestive, one-sided headache accompanied by nausea, vomiting, and pale face. Headache is often brought on by a sense of betrayal and painful memories; seen in anemic women and young girls after a menstrual period. This type of headache is associated with depression and weariness. Fasting, cold bathing, and open air bring relief; consolation, exposure to the sun or heat, noise, and music aggravate the pain. *Remedy: natrum muriaticum.*

  Natrum muriaticum is common salt, sodium chloride. It most benefits people who have a squarish build and who are moody, unhappy, and have frequent, painful memories.

- **Headache caused by overindulgence in food or alcohol or overexposure to the sun or cold wind.** Head pain is often accompanied by nausea, flatulence, vomiting, or a sour or bitter taste in the mouth. Pain is worse in the morning and improves as the day progresses. Headache occurs three hours after a meal. Some people report feeling like they are waiting for vomiting to begin or they wake up with a headache at 3 A.M. Shaking the head is very painful; pain is worse after sleeping or eating. Lying down, wrapping the head, or staying in a warm room may provide some relief. *Remedy: nux vomica,* the "party-lover's" remedy, especially after intake of alcohol, drugs, tobacco, caffeine, or overindulgence of anything.

Nux vomica is prepared from the dried, ripe seeds of the poison-nut tree. This remedy is most effective in thin, quick, active, nervous, irritable individuals. Nux vomica also works well in people who do a lot of mental work.

- *Pain occurs after rich, warm, or fatty foods, such as cheese; also associated with irregular menstrual cycle.* Throbbing accompanies the headache, which is usually felt in the forehead or on one side of the head, although the pain may change location often. A leisurely walk outdoors or in an open area usually offers some relief, even if it causes a chill, but a brisk walk may cause more pain. Cool compresses and cold food or drinks help; warm or overheated rooms make it worse. Mild irritability, weepiness, sweet and loving disposition, emotional sensitivity, and the desire for affection and consolation are characteristic. *Remedy: pulsatilla*

Pulsatilla remedies come from the entire *Pulsatilla nigricans* plant when it is in bloom. This remedy is most beneficial for fair-skinned, fair-haired, plump adults who have a gentle disposition and who tend to be led easily. Females and fair, bright, cheerful children who also tend to be shy and sensitive respond well to pulsatilla.

- *Sharp pain that shoots up through the head, accompanied by sensitivity to noise and light.* Other symptoms include listlessness, constipation, dizziness, nausea, and vomiting. Headache may occur along with menopausal symptoms such as hot flushes and menstruation, especially if scanty. Vigorous exercise, eating, and walking rapidly relieve the pain; smelling food, cold air, and resting, especially in the evening before falling asleep, make the pain worse. *Remedy: sepia.*

Sepia is obtained from the ink of cuttlefish. It works best in individuals who are tall and lean with soft facial features, dark hair, and a yellow complexion. Women going through menopause also respond well.

- *Headache from fasting or skipped meals.* The pain typically begins at back of the head, travels over the top, and settles in one or both eyes, usually the right, and may extend to the face and teeth. The pain can return monthly. Other symptoms include dizziness when looking up, profuse sweating, and hypersensitivity to motion and noise. Sleep offers no relief. The pain is better when the head is wrapped warmly or when lying down. Pain is made worse by damp weather, cold food or drinks, eating, and getting the feet wet. *Remedy: silica.*

Silica is derived from flint and is an essential element for bone development and growth. This is a slow-acting remedy and works best for individuals with a slow metabolism, low stamina, cold hands and feet, and sluggish digestion. It is especially beneficial to children who are small for their age, have delicate skin, large heads, blue eyes, and small hands and feet. Intellectual adults also are helped by silica.

Homeopathy is gaining greater acceptance in the United States as a natural therapy for headache pain as well as many other conditions. When it is used under the guidance of a professional homeopath or other knowledgeable professional, it is a safe, effective, and economical healing technique.

14

DRUGS AND OTHER MEDICAL THERAPIES

Throughout this book, we have explained ways for you to get headache pain relief without the use of drugs or other medical approaches. Sometimes, however, over-the-counter or prescription drugs or other medical therapies may be appropriate for you. Many Americans choose this path, at least part of the time. The National Headache Foundation reported in 1990 that Americans spent more than $4 billion a year on over-the-counter medications for headache. At the same time, more and more people are finding that even if they do use medications occasionally, natural therapies complement the healing process.

There are dozens of drugs for headache pain that work in several different ways to stop or prevent head pain. This chapter contains an overview of the most common over-the-counter and prescription drugs taken for headache pain, as well as a brief explanation of prescribed medical therapies. The drugs are categorized by their primary action; that is, anti-inflammatory, diuretic, beta-blockers, and so on. A complete list of the drugs explained in this chapter appear in the box on pp. 223–25.

All of these drugs may cause unpleasant side effects, and each also has circumstances under which they should not be taken. Because space does not permit us to provide a complete list of these effects or situations for each drug, only the more common ones are given in the following sections. Ask your health-care practitioner or pharmacist for a complete list of side effects and precautions for any drug you take.

As a general rule: If you are currently taking any medication or herbal remedy, consult your physician or pharmacist before starting any new drug, even aspirin. Drug interactions can be serious. Follow package directions for over-the-counter drugs or the advice of your physician or pharmacist for prescription medications.

HEADACHE DRUG THERAPIES*

Over-the-counter analgesics:

- Acetaminophen (Datril and Tylenol; Excedrin, Trigesic, and Vanquish also contain aspirin and caffeine)

Nonsteroidal anti-inflammatory drugs:

- Aspirin[†] (Bayer, Ecotrin, Empirin; Anacin, Anacin Maximum Strength, and Synalgos also contain caffeine)
- Ibuprofen[†] (Motrin, Advil, Nuprin)
- Indomethacin (Indocin)
- Keterolac (Toradol)
- Meclofenamate (Meclomen)
- Naproxen sodium (Anaprox, Aleve,[†] Naprosyn)
- Phenylbutazone (Butazolidin)

Ergot alkaloids:

- Ergotamine tartrate (Bellergal, Cafergot, Wigraine, Ergomar, Ergostat)
- Dihydroergotamine (D.H.E. 45)
- Methysergide (Sansert)

Beta-blockers:

- Atenolol (Tenormin)
- Metoprolol (Lopressor)
- Nadolol (Corgard)
- Propranolol (Inderal)

Calcium-channel blockers:

- Diltiazem (Cardizem)
- Nifedipine (Adalat, Procardia)
- Verapamil (Isoptin, Calan)

Antidepressants/anxiolytics:

- Amitriptyline (Elavil, Endep)
- Buspirone (BuSpar, an antianxiety drug)
- Desipramine (Norpramin)
- Doxepin (Adapin, Sinequan)
- Fluvoxamine (Luvox)
- Fluoxetine (Prozac)
- Imipramine (Tofranil)
- Lithium (Cibalith-S, Eskalith, Lithane, Lithobid)
- Sertraline (Zoloft)
- Trazodone (Desyrel)
- Venlafaxine (Effexor)

Narcotics and narcotic combinations:

- Acetaminophen + caffeine + codeine + butalbital (Fioricet with Codeine)
- Acetaminophen + codeine (Tylenol with Codeine)
- Acetaminophen + oxycodone (Percocet)
- Acetaminophen + hydrocodone (Vicodin)
- Aspirin + caffeine + codeine + butalbital (Fiorinal with Codeine)
- Aspirin + oxycodone (Percodan)
- Butorphanol (Stadol)
- Hydromorphone (Dilaudid)
- Levorphanol (Levo-Dromoran)
- Meperidine (Demerol)
- Morphine (M S Contin, MSIR, Oramorph)
- Nalbuphine (Nubain)
- Pentazocine (Talwin)
- Propoxyphene (Darvon)

Diuretics:

- Acetazolamide (Diamox)
- Furosemide (Lasix)
- Hydrochlorothiazide (HydroDIURIL, Esidrix)
- Spironolactone (Alatone, Aldactone)
- Triamterene (Dyazide, Maxzide)

Corticosteroids:

- Betamethasone (Celestone)
- Dexamethasone (Dexacen, Dexamethasone Intensol, Dexasone, Dexone, and others)

- Prednisone (Deltasone, Orasone, Prednisone Intensol, and others)
- Triamcinolone (Artistocort)

Other Agents

- Acetaminophen + dichloralphenazone + isometheptene mucate (Midrin)
- Capsaicin (Zostrix)
- Chlorpromazine (Thorazine)
- Divalproex (Depakote, Epival)
- Lidocaine (Emla, Xylocaine)
- Oxygen
- Sumatriptan (Imitrex)

*This is only a partial list, representing some of the most common over-the-counter and prescription headache medications. Although some of these drugs have not been approved by the U.S. Food and Drug Administration specifically to treat headache pain, many physicians prescribe them to control headache. Always consult your physician before taking any drugs, and inform all of your physicians about any drugs you are taking.
†Over-the-counter form.

ACETAMINOPHEN

Acetaminophen is a common, over-the-counter pain killer that appears in more than 100 pain medications; for example, Tylenol, Datril, Panadol, Anacin-3, and others. Many people who experience stomach problems when taking aspirin take acetaminophen instead.

SIDE EFFECTS

Although acetaminophen does not cause stomach and intestinal irritation, it is toxic, like aspirin, when high amounts are taken. Other side effects are individual: diarrhea, rash, loss of appetite, painful urination, gastrointestinal upset. Acetaminophen is prescribed for pregnant and breast-feeding women, but it is recommended with caution. Rarely, acetaminophen can cause kidney or liver damage.

NONSTEROIDAL ANTI-INFLAMMATORY DRUGS

Nonsteroidal anti-inflammatory drugs (NSAIDs) are a class of drugs that block the action of inflammatory chemicals in the body, such as prostaglandins, that cause swelling, redness, heat, and pain. Since prostaglandins also help maintain a healthy stomach lining, NSAIDs can block this benefit and therefore can cause stomach and intestinal irritation. Generally, it is recommended that you take NSAIDs with food.

Most of the approximately two dozen NSAIDs on the market are available only by prescription, although aspirin, ibuprofen, and naproxen (Aleve)—the most popular—are available over the counter. Aspirin is the most well known and least costly NSAID. Generally, NSAIDs are equally effective in reducing or eliminating headache pain. People tend to respond better to one or another, but then frequently, the efficacy of that particular drug wears off and after about 2 weeks to 2 months, another agent, even one that did not work the first time, will bring relief.

SIDE EFFECTS

The most common side effects of NSAIDs are intestinal bleeding, peptic ulcers, fluid retention, bruising, kidney and liver damage, headache, joint pain, dizziness, ringing in the ears, and nausea. Most of the bleeding is "occult," not visible in the stool, although if your stool becomes black or like tar, you should have it checked, because this indicates bleeding from the stomach, as blood from the stomach is no longer red by the time it reaches the stool. Blood in the intestines can be mixed with stool, so it also can be hidden. It is possible to lose significant amounts of blood without knowing it and become anemic. Sometimes the bleeding is profuse and dangerous.

COMMON FORMS

The following list contains just a few of the more commonly prescribed and over-the-counter NSAIDs. Your physician may have his or her favorites and may have samples you can try.

- *Aspirin (Anacin, Bayer, Excedrin, Vanquish, and others).* Aspirin is in dozens of over-the-counter pain medications. The enteric form, which has a coating that does not dissolve until the drug reaches the stomach, still can cause stomach or intestinal irritation or bleeding caused by the loss of prostaglandin protection.
- *Ibuprofen (Advil, Medipren, Midol, Motrin, Nuprin, Rufen, and others).* Ibuprofen is available over the counter in 200-mg-strength tablets and is used for tension headaches and migraines. Higher-dose preparations are available by prescription. Do not take ibuprofen if you cannot tolerate aspirin.
- *Indomethacin (Indocin).* Indomethacin is one of the older NSAIDs and is considered one of the more potent in the class. It can also cause serious side effects, such as cardiac failure, hypertension, edema, epilepsy, depression, and tremors, in addition to the adverse effects listed above (under Side Effects). For these reasons, indomethacin is not typically a first choice for headache and is not taken long term if it can be avoided.
- *Keterolac (Toradol).* This drug is a favorite of emergency-room doctors because it is as effective as potent narcotic drugs for treatment of severe migraines. Keterolac is available in both injectable and pill forms, with a maximum

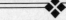

COMBINING DRUGS

Tylenol and aspirin have different mechanisms of action, so if you don't get the relief you want from one, it is better to take the recommended dose of the other agent rather than repeat the dose of the first drug. Do not mix aspirin (which is a nonsteroidal anti-inflammatory drug [NSAID]) with any other NSAID. Therefore:

You can mix: aspirin + acetaminophen
NSAIDS + acetaminophen

But do not mix: aspirin + any other NSAID

injection treatment period of 5 days. Keterolac may cause fluid retention and weight gain, dry mouth, light-headedness, rash, drowsiness, and diarrhea.

- *Meclofenamate (Meclomen).* This medication is often recommended by gynecologists for menstrual cramps and inflammation. Meclofenamate may cause ringing in the ears, fluid retention, hives, dizziness, indigestion, and diarrhea.

- *Naproxen sodium (Aleve, Anaprox, Naprosyn).* Naproxen provides quick relief, in perhaps 20 minutes or less. This drug definitely should be avoided in pregnant and breast-feeding women. Possible side effects include an unpleasant taste and throat irritation or hoarseness. Aleve is available over the counter.

ERGOT ALKALOIDS

Ergot alkaloids typically are used to treat severe headaches, including cluster, migraine, and head pain associated with sexual activity. Each drug has its own specific way of relieving head pain and its own side effects, all of which are explained below.

COMMON FORMS

The following list contains some of the more commonly prescribed ergot alkaloids.

- *Ergotamine tartrate (Ergostat, Cafergot, Wigraine, Bellergal, and others).* Ergotamine tartrate is the most widely used drug as the first line of treatment for moderate to severe migraine and is about 50% effective. It relieves head pain by prompting serotonin to constrict the blood vessels in the head. This action in turn prevents and relieves the pressure caused by expansion of the blood vessels that can cause migraines. Dosages for each of the ergotamine tartrate drugs vary; consult your physician or pharmacist and follow label directions.

    Several formulations of ergotamine are available: the agent alone (Ergomar, Ergostat); combined with caffeine (Wigraine); combined with caffeine, belladonna, and pentobarbital (Cafergot-PB); and combined with belladonna and phenobarbital (Bellergal). Ergotamine can be given orally, by inhalation, sublingually (dissolved under the tongue), or rectally at the first sign of a migraine.

Ergotamine is also effective for the first few bouts of cluster headaches if taken before the predicted time of attack. Up to 80 percent of cluster-headache attacks can be prevented if ergotamine is taken as an aerosol or sublingually just before the attack begins.

Side effects: Common side effects are abdominal or muscle cramps, dizziness, numbness, pain in the arms or legs, diarrhea, malaise, vomiting, drowsiness, jitters, fluctuating heart rate, itching, rebound headache, and complications due to constriction of blood vessels. Ergotamine should not be taken by individuals with high blood pressure, poor circulation, or a history of or high risk of stroke or liver, kidney, or heart disease.

- *Dihydroergotamine (D.H.E. 45).* D.H.E. is the injectable form of ergotamine. It is given intramuscularly when a migraine begins and can be repeated at 8-hour intervals thereafter. To prevent cluster headaches, it can be injected before the attack. Intravenous D.H.E. 45 is the most effective route of administration and can prevent about 80% of cluster-headache attacks. Most physicians shy away from prescribing intravenous D.H.E. 45 because they are not familiar with it and fear its side effects. A nasal form of D.H.E. 45 is scheduled for release soon.

  Side effects: D.H.E. 45 may cause cold hands or feet, nausea, numbness and tingling of the extremities, swollen feet or lower legs, and blisters on the hands or feet.

- *Methysergide (Sansert).* Methysergide is used to prevent migraines and to treat cluster headaches. It is sometimes called an antiserotonin drug because it blocks the inflammatory action of serotonin, thus preventing constriction of the blood vessels in the head and the resulting migraine pain. It is effective in up to 70% of people treated for cluster headaches. For migraines, methysergide eliminates the pain in about 25% of patients and reduces the pain by about 50% in 40–50% of patients.

  Side effects: Methysergide can cause nausea, stomach pain, tired legs, anxiety, thickening of the heart valves (rarely), fibrosis of the lungs or abdominal tissue, and hallucinations. It should not be taken by women who are pregnant or breast-feeding or by people with phlebitis, cellulitis, severe infection, collagen disease, fibrosis, or any type of lung disease. Because it has the potential to cause fibrosis and vascular problems, methysergide's use in migraine patients should be limited to those with severe pain that has not responded to other therapies. It also contains tartrazine, which frequently is associated with causing asthma, hyperactivity, and other symptoms. Patients need to be monitored carefully for side effects and need to take frequent drug "holidays"—periods every 6 months when they stop taking the drug for 1 month.

BETA-BLOCKERS

Beta-blockers (also called beta-adrenergic blockers) are prescribed to prevent migraine attacks. Drugs in this category, which are also prescribed to control blood pressure, block the effect of adrenaline on the cell walls. Since adrenaline causes increased heart rate and constriction of blood vessels, these drugs help lower the heart rate and relax the arteries, resulting in head pain relief.

The most commonly prescribed beta-blockers (atenolol, metoprolol, nadolol, and propranolol) all have similar side effects and similar effectiveness against headache pain (see Side Effects, below). The frequency and intensity of migraine attacks can usually be lessened on lower doses than typically given for blood-pressure control.

SIDE EFFECTS

Beta-blockers can cause cold hands and feet, fatigue, insomnia, asthma, dizziness, depression, mental confusion, heart failure, heart block, rash, itching, hypotension, intestinal upset, and increased cholesterol and triglyceride levels. Never stop taking these drugs suddenly; consult your physician for help in gradually reducing the dosage to avoid serious withdrawal symptoms. Individuals with certain lung, heart, and other conditions should not take beta-blockers. Before taking beta-blockers, be sure the health-care practitioner treating your headaches is aware of all your medical problems and medications, as beta-blockers interact with many other drugs. Because beta-blockers have a direct effect on the heart and lungs and blood chemistry, a medical evaluation is needed before they can be prescribed.

CALCIUM CHANNEL BLOCKERS

Calcium channel blockers prohibit calcium from passing through vessel cell walls and thus help prevent muscle contractions of the vessel walls. Calcium channel blockers are used to treat both migraines and cluster headaches and may be better tolerated than beta-blockers. The most common calcium channel blockers used to treat headache pain include diltiazem, nifedipine, and verapamil.

SIDE EFFECTS

Calcium channel blockers can cause constipation, depression, dizziness, hypotension, allergic reactions, fluid retention, fatigue, and impotence. Calcium channel blockers can also adversely affect the heart; therefore, a cardiac evaluation is recommended before treatment begins.

ANTIDEPRESSANTS

Even without any signs of depression, antidepressants have proven to be effective in reducing many kinds of pain, including head pain, and at relatively low doses—sometimes as low as $1/50$ of the dosage for depression. Several categories of antidepressants are prescribed for headache.

TRICYCLIC ANTIDEPRESSANTS

The four drugs frequently prescribed for headache pain in this category include amitriptyline, doxepin, desipramine, and imipramine. All are similarly effective and have side effects in common. They relieve pain by affecting the part of the brain that controls pain signals between nerve cells, and they can also help you sleep.

Side effects: Tricyclic antidepressants can cause morning drowsiness, dry mouth, nausea, cardiac arrhythmias, flushing, weight gain, headache, rash, and increased perspiration. Dry mouth, dizziness, and constipation can frequently be alleviated with the choline found in lecithin, which is available at health-food stores.

SEROTONIN-REUPTAKE-INHIBITOR AND SIMILAR ANTIDEPRESSANTS

Generally, the drugs in the category of serotonin-reuptake-inhibitor (SRI) (fluoxetine, fluvoxamine, paroxetine, sertraline, and trazodone) relieve headache pain by restoring the serotonin level in the brain to normal. A sixth, venlafaxine, works on serotonin as well as other chemical levels in the brain. Overall, the SRIs may be most beneficial because they help lift depression and energize you to make healthful changes in your life.

You may need to remain on an SRI for more than 1 month to see the preventive effect for headache. Some people improve dramatically in terms of stress, depression, insomnia, and various behavioral problems when taking SRIs. However, it is very hard to stop taking these drugs, and you should do so only under the supervision of your physician. As yet, the drugs' long-term effects and impact on personal growth are not clear.

Side effects: Overall, these drugs have less sedative and cardiovascular impact than do tricyclics. Possible side effects include drowsiness, dizziness, tremor, headache, chills, jaw pain, anxiety, insomnia, nausea, vomiting, diarrhea, agitation, bradycardia, fatigue, sexual dysfunction, sweating, dry mouth, lightheadedness, constipation, confusion or disorientation, seizures, and hallucinations.

LITHIUM

Another antidepressant drug sometimes prescribed for chronic cluster headaches is lithium (Cibalith-S, Eskalith, Lithane, Lithobid). To relieve headache pain, lithium may correct imbalances in the brain's transmission of pain signals. It is associated with inconsistent results and many side effects. If manic depression is a factor, however, it may be the drug of choice for you.

Side effects: Lithium can cause diarrhea, tremors, excessive urination, hypothyroidism, nausea, drowsiness, blurred vision, metallic taste, uncontrollable movements called extrapyramidal symptoms, dry mouth, seizures, and hypotension. Frequent blood tests are necessary to check blood levels.

BUSPIRONE

For chronic headaches associated with anxiety, buspirone (BuSpar) may be your choice. It relieves pain by affecting the transmission of nerve impulses in the brain.

Side effects: Buspirone can cause sedation, dizziness, nausea, headache, nervousness, dream disturbances, and nonspecific chest pain.

NARCOTIC ANALGESICS

Narcotic analgesics depress pain signals in the brain and spinal cord, thus relieving headache pain. These drugs are addictive, and physicians usually avoid prescribing them except for severe or sudden, short-lived head pain. Some narcotics are single agents; others are combined with analgesics or a barbiturate (see box on pp. 223–25).

SIDE EFFECTS

Narcotic analgesics can cause sedation, dizziness, sweating, dry mouth, nausea, vomiting, constipation, urinary retention, hypotension, rash, convulsions, allergy, and respiratory depression. People who have asthma, gastritis, or impaired renal, thyroid, or liver function; who are age 65 or older; or who have increased intracranial pressure should avoid narcotic analgesics.

DIURETICS

Diuretics reduce blood pressure by increasing the amount of salt released into the urine by the kidneys. Along with the salt, the kidneys also release water and potassium, unless the diuretic specifically is "potassium-sparing." Diuretics are used to treat head pain caused by increased fluid pressure in the head—for example, altitude-related headache, premenstrual headache caused by hormone-induced water retention, and benign intra-cranial headache. The most common diuretics prescribed for headache pain include acetazolamide, furosemide, hydrochloro-thiazide, spironolactone, and triamterene. The latter two are potassium-sparing.

SIDE EFFECTS

Diuretics can cause hypotension, drowsiness, muscle cramps, headache, confusion, gastrointestinal distress, weakness, ringing in the ears, and depression. In otherwise healthy women, herbal diuretics generally can relieve the water retention that accompa-nies premenstrual syndrome.

CORTICOSTEROIDS

Corticosteroids relieve headache pain by preventing inflamma-tion of the tissues in the head and neck. These drugs are usually reserved for severe cases of headache due to inflammation, such as in temporal arteritis or head pain caused by high altitudes. Corticosteroids commonly prescribed for headache pain include betamethasone, dexamethasone, prednisone, and triamcinolone. In headache caused by temporal arteritis (see Chapter 5), they are given to suppress inflammation of the temporal artery. In-jectable steroids are administered to prevent swelling in the head in very high altitudes. Some physicians also inject steroids to treat trigger points in muscle-tension headache. Injectable ho-meopathic remedies are an alternative (see Chapter 13). In rare cases, steroidal drugs are given to patients with migraine who have not obtained relief from other therapies.

SIDE EFFECTS

Corticosteroids can cause acne, thirst, indigestion, nausea, un-pleasant taste, cough, hoarseness, high blood pressure, swelling, bruising, abnormal weight gain, local dying (necrosis) of under-lying tissue when given by injection, psychological disturbances, adverse effects on blood sugar and key electrolytes, ulcers, headache, and suppression of the immune system, which can lead to infections. Corticosteroids should not be taken by people who have tuberculosis, cirrhosis, viral diseases such as herpes, peptic ulcer, hypothyroidism, renal insufficiency, or ulcerative colitis.

OTHER DRUGS

CAPSAICIN (ZOSTRIX, AMONG OTHERS)

Capsaicin, a derivative of red hot chili peppers, is a new treatment for cluster headaches, as well as for arthritis, postoperative pain, shingles, and other painful conditions. Capsaicin is the active ingredient in this over-the-counter, topical cream that has shown good success in treating cluster headache. Capsaicin stimulates an increase in the amount of substance P, a neurotransmitter that relays pain messages to the brain. Repeated applications of capsaicin to a particular spot eventually depletes the supply of substance P at that location. This appears to explain why reports from early studies show a significant improvement in pain after patients with cluster headaches apply a small amount of the cream once or twice a day into the nostril on the affected side. Dr. Alan Rapoport, director of The New England Center for Headache in Stamford, Connecticut, participated in a study of cluster headache patients and believes capsaicin may have application to migraine patients as well.

Side effects: Capsaicin may cause stinging or burning at the application site.

CHLORPROMAZINE (THORAZINE)

The antipsychotic chlorpromazine is recommended only for severe, incapacitating headache unmanageable by other means. It relieves pain by suppressing nerve transmission in parts of the brain.

Side effects: Chlorpromazine can cause irreversible and reversible central nervous system damage, extreme drowsiness, hypotension, cardiovascular problems, and others. Chlorpromazine has many drug interactions. Avoid this drug if also taking clonidine, propranolol, guanethidine, or antidiabetic drugs.

DIVALPROEX (DEPAKOTE, EPIVAL)

Although divalproex is used primarily to treat epilepsy, it is also an effective treatment for migraine. One study shows that the drug reduces the frequency of migraine by about $1/2$ in 50 percent of people who try it. Divalproex relieves pain by inhibiting nerve transmissions in part of the brain. It is recommended for people with frequent headaches and is considered safe for long-term use.

Side effects: Divalproex can cause nausea, menstrual irregularities, lethargy, drowsiness, headache, dizziness, unsteadiness, confusion, indigestion, and stomach cramps.

LIDOCAINE (XYLOCAINE, EMLA)

The anesthetic agent lidocaine can be used to treat cluster headache, trigeminal neuralgia, and headache associated with head trauma. It is available in several formulations. As drops, gel, or spray, it can be put into the nostril on the affected side during a cluster-headache attack to help numb the nerve endings and ease the pain. It also is used in nerve blocks for trigeminal neuralgia and headache associated with head trauma (see Medical and Surgical Interventions, in this chapter). Lidocaine and procaine (Novocain, Ardecaine, among others) are effective when injected into trigger points for muscle-tension headache. Homeopathic injections are an alternative.

Side effects: Lidocaine can cause sleepiness, stupor, slurred speech, anxiety, depression, numbness, muscle twitching, seizures, low blood pressure, ringing in the ears, blurred or double vision, rash, and severe allergic reactions.

MIDRIN

Midrin is a combination drug (acetaminophen, dichloralphenazone—a mild, nonaddicting sedative—and isometheptene mucate, a blood-vessel constrictor) used for mild to moderate pain. It relieves pain by causing the blood vessels in the head to constrict. Midrin is well tolerated by young children and by the elderly.

Side effects: Midrin can cause fatigue, mild stomach upset, light-headedness, and increased blood pressure.

SUMATRIPTAN

Sumatriptan (Imitrex) causes dilated blood vessels in the head to constrict and also reduces the nausea, vomiting, and sensitivity to light that occur with migraines. It also is very effective for treatment of cluster headaches. Studies show migraine relief within an hour, even as quickly as 15 minutes, in up to 75 percent of patients, compared with only 25 percent of patients who obtained relief from placebos. Sumatriptan is available as an injectable form and in tablets. If taken as an injection, a repeat injection is not recommended until the beginning of the next episode of pain, as a follow-up dose does not appear to prevent recurrence.

Side effects: Sumatriptan can cause dizziness, flushing, nausea, and vomiting. Sumatriptan should not be taken if you have definite or possible ischemic heart disease, especially Prinzmetal's angina, uncontrolled hypertension, or if you are also taking ergotamines. The caution against use in people with possible heart problems arises from the occurrence of anginalike chest pain in 3 to 5 percent of patients who get a sumatriptan injection. Caution is recommended for sumatriptan use in postmenopausal women, men older than 50, and individuals with a high risk of heart disease, hypertension, a high cholesterol level, obesity, tobacco use, and Reynaud's disease or vascular disease.

A FINAL WORD ON MEDICATIONS

The drug information provided in this chapter is by no means complete, and you are urged to keep the lines of communication open with your health-care provider about all the medications you take. All prescription medications, especially narcotics, may provide dramatic, even rapid relief of your headache pain, yet the reprieve is often temporary, lasting a few days, weeks, or months before the pain returns. The pain may shift to your neck or lower back, or there may be a side effect to a medicine that demands relief. Thus, drugs, while having a place in headache treatment, rarely provide permanent relief.

MEDICAL AND SURGICAL INTERVENTIONS

Occasionally, headache pain does not respond adequately to either natural or pharmaceutical treatments; perhaps an accompanying medical condition makes it necessary to use another approach. People who have chronic, severe headaches, such as cluster or trigeminal neuralgia with debilitating pain, and whose condition does not respond to other treatments may choose to receive injections of lidocaine and corticosteroids, which can be given to deaden the impulses transmitting pain messages along specific nerves to the brain (see Chapter 13, for injectable homeopathic remedies). One common technique for such persistent, severe headache pain is to inject lidocaine, along with betamethasone or another corticosteroid, directly into the occipital nerve, which is located in the back of the head. The steroid reduces local inflammation. Side effects from such injections are rare. Corticosteroid injections can be made into the spine also. These procedures can be done in the doctor's office.

In those rare cases in which headache is caused by a tumor or other lesion on the brain, surgical removal of the growth is common. In headache caused by excess fluid in the brain, as in benign intracranial hypertension (see Chapter 5), lumbar puncture may be performed to relieve the pressure on the brain. Lumbar puncture relieves the pain for most individuals with this type of headache.

Another procedure for severe, persistent headache pain is radio frequency surgery, in which physicians use radio waves to interfere with the pain signals that are being transmitted to the brain. This procedure can be done on an outpatient basis and can be repeated if the pain returns.

A noninvasive medical therapy for many people who suffer from cluster headache is oxygen therapy. Many people with cluster headache find it useful to have an oxygen tank and mask available at home or work so they can put on the mask as soon as the first signs of an attack appear. Inhalation of 100 percent oxygen through a tight-fitting mask for 10 to 15 minutes can eliminate cluster headache pain in about 75 percent of people who use this therapy. In a study of 52 patients who each treated 10 episodes of cluster headache with oxygen, 75 percent of those with acute cluster headache obtained relief, while a higher percentage of those with episodic cluster headache reported some relief.

For many people, drugs or other medical therapies have been the only way they have treated their headache. We believe the natural healing approach is best in most cases. Occasionally, however, you may need drugs or medical procedures to relieve your pain, or you may opt to try natural therapies while tapering off drug use. This chapter has offered you an overview of the medical options available to you.

THE WHOLE PICTURE

Welcome to the end of this book and hopefully to the end of, or a significant reduction in, your headache pain. We have shown you that when it comes to treating your head pain, you have options beyond conventional medical treatment. Have you made yourself some herbal tea, tried self-hypnosis, dabbled with meditation, or received manual healing from an osteopath? Have you made a commitment to add a relaxing movement routine to your daily morning schedule or to investigate some nutritional supplements and a healthier eating plan? Whatever decisions you have made, you deserve to feel better.

Feeling good also means acting responsibly. That's why we strongly recommend that before you begin any therapy program, you see your physician to rule out the slight possibility that your headache pain has an underlying medical cause.

Although the natural therapies presented in this book have been offered with the hope they will provide you with relief from your headache pain, you will likely find that they also give you other bonuses as well: reduced stress, more vitality, increased alertness, better circulation, a sense of calm, and a feeling that *you* have control over your pain. This is the most important gift we can offer you: tools to help you take more control of your life and your pain so you can more fully enjoy the former and eliminate the latter.

NOTES

CHAPTER 1

Eisenberg, David M. et al. "Unconventional Medicine in the United States." *New England Journal of Medicine* 328:246–252, 1993.

Lindlahr, Henry. *Philosophy of Natural Therapeutics.* Chicago: Lindlahr Publishing, 1919.

National Headache Foundation. National Foundation fact sheet, Chicago, 1990.

CHAPTER 2

Gallagher, R. M. "Medical Management of Acute Tension-Type Headache Episodes. In *Headache: Diagnosis and Treatment*, ed. C. David Tollison and Robert S. Kunkel. Baltimore: Williams & Wilkins, 1992, pp. 143–150.

Kudrow, L. "Cluster Headache." In *Migraine: Clinical, Therapeutic, Conceptual and Research Aspects*, ed. J. N. Blau. London: Chapman and Hall, 1987, pp. 113–132.

Steinmetzer, Robert V. "Differential Diagnosis and Related Medical Conditions." In *Headache: Diagnosis and Treatment*, ed. C. David Tollison and Robert S. Kunkel. Baltimore: Williams & Wilkins, 1992, pp. 19–22.

Tollison, C. David. "Nature and Magnitude of Headache." In *Headache: Diagnosis and Treatment*, ed. C. David Tollison and Robert S. Kunkel. Baltimore: Williams & Wilkins, 1992, pp. 3–8.

CHAPTER 3

Buxbaum, Jerome, and Norbert Myslinski. "Headache Associated with Temporomandibular Dysfunction." In *Headache: Diagnosis and Treatment*, ed. C. David Tollison and Robert S. Kunkel. Baltimore: Williams & Wilkins, 1992, pp. 257–264.

Committee on Classification of Headache of the National Institute of Neurological Diseases and Blindness. "Classification of Headache." *Journal of the American Medical Association* 179:717–718, 1962.

Goddard, Greg, D.D.S. *The Jaw Connection: The Overlooked Diagnosis.* Santa Fe, NM: Aurora Press, 1991, p. 10.

Kahn, Ada. *Headaches.* New York: American Family Health Institute, 1983, p. 36.

Lance, James W. *Mechanism and Management of Headache,* 5th ed. London: Butterworth-Heinemann, 1993, p. 148.

Travell, J. G., and D. G. Simons. *Myofascial Pain and Dysfunction: The Trigger Point Manual.* Baltimore: Williams & Wilkins, 1983, pp. 184–206.

Weeks, V. D., and J. Travell. "Postural Vertigo Due to Trigger Areas in the Sternocleidomastoid Muscle." *Journal of Pediatrics* 47:315–327, 1955.

CHAPTER 4

Graham, J. R. "Cluster Headache." *Headache* 11:175–185, 1972.

Hoffert, Marvin. "Treatment of Migraine: A New Era." *American Family Physician* 49:633–638, 1994.

Kudrow, L. *Cluster Headache Mechanisms and Management.* Oxford: Oxford University Press, 1980, pp. 10–19.

Lance, J. W., and M. Anthony. "Some Clinical Aspect of Migraine. A Prospective Survey of 500 Patients." *Archives of Neurology* 15:356–361, 1966.

Life magazine, February 1994, p. 76.

Murray, Michael T., and Joseph L. Pizzorne. *Encyclopedia of Natural Medicine.* Rocklin, CA: Prima Publishing, 1991, pp. 410*ff.*

Rothner, A. David. "Headache in a Pediatric Population." In *Headache: Diagnosis and Treatment,* ed. C. David Tollison and Robert S. Kunkel. Baltimore: Williams & Wilkins, 1992, pp. 271–280.

Selby, G., and J. W. Lance. "Observations on 500 Cases of Migraine and Allied Vascular Headache." *Journal of Neurology, Neurosurgery and Psychiatry* 23:23–32, 1960.

Theiss, Barbara, and Peter Theiss. "Healing Herbs for Headaches." In *The Family Herbal.* Rochester, VT: Healing Arts Press, 1989, p. 139.

Welch, K. M. A., M.D. "Helping Patients Fend Off Migraine Attacks." *Emergency Medicine* 27:45–64, 1995.

CHAPTER 5

Bergkvist, L. et al. "The Risk of Breast Cancer After Estrogen and Estrogen-Progestin Replacement." *New England Journal of Medicine* 321:293–297, 1989.

Durcan, F. J. et al. "The Incidence of Pseudotumor Cerebri: Population Studies in Iowa and Louisiana." *Archives of Neurology* 45:874–877, 1988.

Epstein, M. T. et al. "Migraine and Reproductive Hormones Throughout the Menstrual Cycle." *Lancet* ii:543–548, 1975.

Freenblatt, R. B., and D. W. Bruneteau. "Menopausal Headache—Psychogenic or Metabolic?" *Journal of the American Geriatric Society* 283:186–190, 1974.

Hill, Larry M., and Glen Hastings. "Carotidynia: A Pain Syndrome." *Journal of Family Practice* 39:71–75, 1994.

Hudson, Tori. "Migraine Headaches in Women and Hormonal Influences." *Townsend Letter for Doctors* February/March:249, 1994.

Iansek, R. "Cervical Spondylosis and Headaches." *Clinical and Experimental Neurology* May:175–178, 1982.

Isselbacher, Kurt J. et al., eds. *Harrison's Principles of Internal Medicine*, 13th ed. New York: McGraw-Hill, 1994, p. 787.

Jaff, Michael R., and Glen D. Solomon. "Headaches Associated with Medical Diseases." In *Headache: Diagnosis and Treatment*, ed. C. David Tollison and Robert S. Kunkel. Baltimore: Williams & Wilkins, 1992, pp. 233–238.

Kudrow, L. "The Relationship of Headache Frequency to Hormone Dose in Migraine." *Headache* 15:36–349, 1975.

Lance, James. *Mechanism and Management of Headache*. London: Butterworth-Heineman, 1993.

Lee, John R., M.D. *Natural Progesterone: The Multiple Roles of a Remarkable Hormone*. BLL Publishing, 1994, pp. 50ff.

Margolis, Simeon, ed. *The Johns Hopkins Medical Handbook*. New York: Rebus, 1992, p. 130.

Mason, V. "Switch Pills for Headaches and Mood Swing, but Not Weight Gain, Say Readers." *Contraceptive Technology Update* 14:133–136, 1993.

Messina, Mike, and Virginia Messina. *The Simple Soybean and Your Health*. Garden City, NY: Avery Publishing Group, 1994.

Meyer, John Stirling, and Jun Kawamura. "Cerebral Vascular Disease and Headache." In *The Practicing Physician's Approach to Headache*, 5th ed., ed. Seymour Diamond. Baltimore: Williams & Wilkins, 1992, p. 167.

Peterson, P. K. et al. "A Controlled Trial of Intravenous Immunoglobulin G in Chronic Fatigue Syndrome." *American Journal of Medicine* 89:554–560, 1990.

Pizzorno, Joseph, and Michael T. Murray. *A Textbook of Natural Medicine*. Seattle: Jon Bastyr College Publications, 1988, VI;MS-5.

Prior, J. C. et al. "Progesterone and the Prevention of Osteoporosis." *Canadian Journal of Obstetrics/Gynecology and Women's Health Care* 3:178–184, 1991.

Ratinahirana, H. et al. "Migraine and Pregnancy: A Prospective Study in 703 Women After Delivery." *Neurology* 40:437, 1990.

Ryan, R. E. "A Controlled Study of the Effect of Oral Contraceptives on Migraine." *Headache* 17:250-252, 1978.

Schon, F., and J. N. Blau. "Post-epileptic Headache and Migraine." *Journal of Neurology, Neurosurgery and Psychiatry* 50:1148–1152, 1987.

Silberstein, S. D. "Headaches and Women: Treatment of the Pregnant and Lactating Migraineur." *Headache* 33:533–540, 1993.

Speroff, Leon. *Clinical Gynecological Endocrinology and Infertility*, 5th ed. Baltimore: Williams & Wilkins, 1994.

Whitty, C. W. M., and J. M. Hockaday. "Migraine: A Follow-up Study of 92 Patients." *British Medical Journal* 1:735–736, 1986.

Whitty, C. W. M. et al. "The Effect of Oral Contraceptives on Migraine." *Lancet* i:856–859, 1966.

CHAPTER 6

Becker, W. J. "Chronic Daily Headache and Analgesic Overuse." *Canadian Journal of Continuing Medical Education* August:77–83, 1994.

de Belleroche, J. et al. "Erythrocyte Choline Concentrations and Cluster Headache." *British Medical Journal* 288:268–270, 1984.

derBergh, V. V. et al. "Trigger Factors in Migraine: A Study Conducted by the Belgian Migraine Society." *Headache* 27:191–196, 1987.

Harrison, D. P. "Copper As a Factor in the Dietary Precipitation of Migraine." *Headache* 26:248–250, 1986.

Jankovic. "Benign Coital Cephalalgia. Differential Diagnosis and Treatment." *Archives of Neurology* 38:710–712, 1981.

Koehler, S. M. "The Effect of Aspartame on Migraine Headache." *Headache* 28:10–14, 1988.

Lance, J. W. "Headaches Related to Sexual Activity." *Journal of Neurology, Neurosurgery and Psychiatry* 39:1226–1230, 1976.

Lipton, R. B. "Aspartame as a Dietary Trigger of Headache." *Headache* 29:90–99, 1989.

Murray, Michael T. *Natural Alternatives to Over-the-Counter and Prescription Drugs.* New York: William Morrow, 1994, p. 192.

Murray, Michael T., and Joseph E. Pizzorno. *Encyclopedia of Natural Medicine.* Rocklin, CA: Prima Publishing, 1991, pp. 305–321, 410–421.

New England Journal of Medicine 317:1181–1185, 1987.

Ramadan, N. M. et al. "Low Brain Magnesium in Migraine." *Headache* 29:590–593, 1989.

Raskin, N. H. "Headache: An Overview." In *Headache,* 1st ed. New York: Churchill Livingstone, 1988, pp. 16-17.

Saper, J. R. "Daily Chronic Headache." *Neurologic Clinics* 8:891–901, 1990.

Schiffman, Susan S. et al. "Aspartame and Susceptibility to Headache."

Solomon, Seymour. *The Headache Book.* Yonkers, NY: Consumer Reports Books, 1991, p. 23.

Somer, Elizabeth. *The Essential Guide to Vitamins and Minerals.* New York: Harper Perennial, 1992, p. 58.

Soriani, S. et al. "Serum and Red Blood Cell Migraine Levels in Juvenile Migraine Patients." *Headache* 35:14–16, 1995.

Soriani, S. et al. "Magnesium Lower in Migraine Patients." *Headache* 34:160–165, 1994.

Swanson, D. R. "Migraine and Magnesium: Eleven Neglected Connections." *Perspectives in Biology and Medicine* 31:526–557, 1988.

Tollison, C. D., and R. S. Kunkel, eds. *Headache: Diagnosis and Treatment.* Baltimore: Williams & Wilkins, 1992, p. 303.

van den Eeden, S. K. et al. "Aspartame Ingestion and Headaches: A Randomized Crossover Trial." *Neurology* 44:1787–1793, 1994.

CHAPTER 7

Achterberg, Jeanne, Ph.D. Adapted from *Rituals of Healing: Using Imagery for Health and Wellness.* New York: Bantam Books, 1994, pp. 120–122.

Benson, Herbert, M.D. *The Wellness Book.* New York: Carol Publishing Group, 1992, p. 35.

Blanchard, E. B., and F. Andrasik. "Psychological Assessment and Treatment of Headache: Recent Developments and Emerging Issues." *Journal of Consulting and Clinical Psychology* 50:859–879, 1982.

Blanchard, E. B., and F. Andrasik. "Biofeedback Treatment of Vascular Head-
    ache." In *Biofeedback: Studies in Clinical Efficacy*, ed. J. P. Hatch et al. New
    York: Plenum Press, 1987, pp. 1–79.
The Institute for Bioenergetic Analysis, 144 E. 36th St., New York, NY 10016;
    from a syllabus prepared by Dr. Maas.
Kittredge, Mary. *Pain*. New York: Chelsea House Publishers, 1992, p. 81.
Monte, Tom et al. *World Medicine: The East West Guide to Healing Your Body*. New
    York: Jeremy Tarcher, 1993, p. 166.
Olness, Karen, M.D. "Hypnosis: The Power of Attention." In *Mind/Body Medi-
    cine*. New York: Consumer Reports Books, 1993, pp. 301–313.
Rossman, Martin L., M.D. "Imagery: Learning to Use the Mind's Eye." In
    Mind/Body Medicine. New York: Consumer Reports Books, 1993, pp. 291–
    300.
Schwartz, Mark S., and Nancy M. Schwartz. "Biofeedback: Using the Body's
    Signals." In *Mind/Body Medicine*. New York: Consumer Reports Books,
    1993, pp. 301–313.
Weil, Andrew, M.D. *Natural Health, Natural Medicine*. Boston: Houghton
    Mifflin, 1990, p. 126.

CHAPTER 8

Cowles, Jane. *Pain Relief*. New York: MasterMedia Ltd., 1993, p. 103.
Trevelyan, Joanna. "Alexander Technique." *Nursing Times* 89:50–52, 1993.

CHAPTER 9

Hansen, P. E., and J. H. Hansen. "Acupuncture Treatment of Chronic Tension
    Headache: A Controlled Cross-over Trial. *Cephalgia* 5:137–142, 1985.
Keller, E., and V. M. Bzdek. "Effects of Therapeutic Touch on Tension Head-
    ache Pain." *Nursing Research* 35:101–106, 1986.
Loh, L. et al. "Acupuncture Versus Medial Treatment for Migraine and Muscle
    Tension Headaches." *Journal of Neurology, Neurosurgery and Psychiatry*
    47:333–337, 1984.
Prevention magazine editors. *Hands-On Healing*. Emmaus, PA: Rodale Press,
    1993, p. 319.
Sjolund, B. et al. "Increased Cerebrospinal Fluid Levels of Endorphins After
    Electroacupuncture." *Acta Physiological Scandinavia* 100:382–384, 1977.
Ulett, George A. "Acupuncture." In *Headache: Diagnosis and Treatment*, ed. C.
    David Tollison and Robert S. Kunkel. Baltimore: Williams & Wilkins, 1992,
    pp. 391–397.
Vincent, C. A. "The Treatment of Tension Headache by Acupuncture: A Con-
    trolled Single-Case Design with Time Series Analysis. *Journal of Psychoso-
    matic Research* 35:553–561, 1990.

CHAPTER 10

Feltman, John, ed., and *Prevention* magazine editors. *Hands-On Healing*. Em-
    maus, PA: Rodale Press, 1992, p. 146.

Prevention magazine editors. *The Prevention Pain-Relief System.* Emmaus, PA: Rodale Press, 1992, p. 526.

Prudden, Bonnie. *Pain-Erasure: The Bonnie Prudden Way.* New York: Ballantine Books, 1980, pp. 46–47.

CHAPTER 11

Carper, Jean. *Food—Your Miracle Medicine.* New York: Harper Collins, 1993, p. 321.

Egger, J. "Is Migraine Food Allergy? A Double-Blind Controlled Trial of Oligoantigenic Diet Treatment." *Lancet* 2:865–869, 1983.

Glueck, C. J. et al. "Amelioration of Severe Migraine with Omega-3 Fatty Acids." *American Journal of Clinical Nutrition* 43:710, 1986.

Hendler, Sheldon Saul. *The Doctors' Vitamin and Mineral Encyclopedia.* New York: Simon & Schuster, 1990, pp. 39ff., 157–164.

Hitzemann, R. J. Research conducted at State University of New York, Stony Brook, 1986; Charles Glueck. Research conducted at University of Cincinnati College of Medicine, 1986.

Jarvis, D. C. *Folk Medicine.* New York: Fawcett, Crest Book, 1973, pp. 124–126.

Jones, A., and C. Harrop. "Study of Migraine and the Study of Attacks in Industry." *Journal of Internal Medicine* 8:321–325, 1980.

Lu, Henry C. *Chinese System of Food Cures.* New York: Sterling Publishing, pp. 48, 57–59, 60, 95, 97, 1986.

Gallai, V. et al. "Magnesium Content of Mononuclear Blood Cells in Migraine Patients." *Headache* 34:160-165, 1994.

National Headache Foundation. National Headache Foundation fact sheet, Chicago, 1990.

"Patients with Migraine May Benefit from Magnesium Supplements." *Headache* 33:135–138, 1993.

Trattler, Ross. *Better Health Through Natural Healing.* New York: McGraw-Hill, 1988, pp. 314–315.

Werbach, Melvyn, M.D. *Healing with Food.* New York: Harper Collins, 1993, pp. 255–261, 293–301.

Whitaker, Julian, M.D. *Dr. Whitaker's Guide to Natural Healing.* Rocklin, CA: Prima Publishing, 1995, pp. 257–260.

CHAPTER 12

Armstrong, F. "Scenting Relief." *Nursing Times* 87:52–54, 1991.

Fischer-Rizzi, Susanne. *Complete Aromatherapy Handbook.* Translated from German. New York: Sterling Publishing, 1990, p. 165.

Hewitt, Dawn. "Massage with Lavender Oil Lowered Tension." *Nursing Times* 88:25, 1992.

Johnson, E. S. et al. "Efficacy of Feverfew As Prophylactic Treatment of Migraine." *British Medical Journal* 291:569–573, 1985.

Murphy, J. J. et al. "Randomized Double-Blind Placebo-Controlled Trial of Feverfew in Migraine Prevention." *Lancet* ii:189–192, 1988.

Murray, Michael T., N.D. *Natural Alternatives to Over-the-Counter and Prescription Drugs.* New York: William Morrow, 1994, p. 287.

Prevention magazine editors. *The Complete Book of Natural and Medicinal Cures.* Emmaus, PA: Rodale Press, 1994.

Sherman, John A., N.D. *The Complete Botanical Prescriber.* Compiled by John A. Sherman, N.D., 1993.

Tierra, Michael, N.D. *Planetary Herbology.* Twin Lakes, WI: Lotus Press, 1988.

Tierra, Michael, N.D. *The Way of Herbs.* New York: Simon & Schuster, 1990.

Trevelyan, Joanna. "Aromatherapy." *Nursing Times* 89:38–40, 1993.

CHAPTER 13

British Medical Journal June 1986.

Cummings, Stephen, and Dana Ullman. *Everybody's Guide to Homeopathic Medicine.* Los Angeles: Jeremy P. Tarcher, 1991.

Lockie, Andrew. *The Home Guide to Homeopathy.* New York: Simon & Schuster, 1989; 1993, pp. 133–134.

Rose, Barry. *The Family Health Guide to Homeopathy.* Berkeley, CA: Celestrial Arts, 1992.

Ullman, Dana. *Homeopathy: Medicine for the 21st Century.* Berkeley, CA: North Atlantic Books, pp. 110, 114, 115, 117, 1988.

Weiner, Michael. *The Complete Book of Homeopathy.* Garden City, NY: Avery Publishing Group, 1989.

Weinstein, Corey, and Nancy Bruning. *Healing Homeopathic Remedies.* New York: Dell Publishing, 1996.

CHAPTER 14

Archives of Neurology March 1995.

Cicala, R. S., and J. R. Jernigan. "Nerve Blocks and Invasive Therapies." In *Headache: Diagnosis and Treatment,* ed. C. David Tollison and Robert S. Kunkel. Baltimore: Williams & Wilkins, 1992, p. 362.

Curran, D. A. et al. "Methysergide." *Research and Clinical Studies in Headache* 1:74–122, 1967.

Houghton, L. A. et al. "Is Chest Pain after Sumatriptan Oesophageal in Origin?" *Lancet* 344:985–986, 1994.

Kudrow, L. "Response of Cluster Headache Attacks to Oxygen Inhalation." *Headache* 21:1–4, 1981.

McKenna, M. P. "Cluster Headache." *American Family Physician* 37:173–178, 1988.

Modern Medicine 62:26, 1994,

National Headache Foundation, National Headache Foundation fact sheet, Chicago, 1990.

Tollison, C. D., and J. W. Tollison. *Headache: A Multimodel Program for Relief.* New York: Sterling Publishing, p. 11, 1982.

USA Today 23 August, 1994, "Taking the Fire Out of Pain with Essence of Chile Pepper."

Welch, K. M. A. "Helping Patients Fend Off Migraine Attacks." *Emergency Medicine* 27:45–64, 1995.

APPENDIX I
Where to Find Information and Health-Care Professionals

Searching for a natural therapy practitioner?
- Look in the yellow pages of the telephone book.
- Get referrals from friends and family.
- Get referrals from your physician.
- Contact the organizations listed below. Many also have literature and other helpful information available. Ask questions! Be an informed consumer. Some organizations will take requests for written information over the telephone; others prefer that you send a stamped, self-addressed envelope (SASE—business size).

GENERAL INFORMATION

American Academy of Osteopathy
3500 DePauw Blvd.
Indianapolis, IN 46268
(317) 879-1881

American Holistic Medical Association
433 Front St.
Catasauqua, PA 18032
(610) 433-2448

American Association of Naturopathic Physicians
P.O. Box 2579
Kirkland, WA 98083-2579
(206) 827-6035

WHAT IS A NATUROPATH?
Naturopaths are the only licensed primary health-care practitioners who receive comprehensive training in therapeutic diets and preventive nutrition. Naturopaths can train at one of the three naturopathic medical schools in the United States, where they complete a four-year doctoral program that leads to the doctor of naturopathic medicine (N.D.) degree. Preadmission requirements for these schools are similar to those of conventional medical schools.

Naturopathic training includes 128 classroom and clinic hours in diet, disease, and therapeutic diets; most medical schools do not address these areas. They also spend 1,300 hours of internship in diet and disease; medical internships do not normally include this training. Another 150 hours of classroom and clinic time is spent in behavior-oriented counseling. This counseling training is instrumental in the practice of naturopathy. (Source: American Association of Naturopathic Physicians)

American Council for Headache Education
875 Kings Highway, Suite 200
West Deptford, NJ 08096
(800) 255-2243
Focuses on education and research about headache.

American Chronic Pain Association
P.O. Box 850
Rocklin, CA 95677
(916) 632-0922
Provides useful information and other services (newsletter, workbooks) about
    chronic pain, headache included.

Complementary Medicine Networking and Referral Service
4649 Malvern
Tucson, AZ 85711
(520) 323-6291
Answers questions; gives referrals to holistic and/or general physicians.

ACUPRESSURE AND ACUPUNCTURE

American Oriental Bodywork Association
6801 Jericho Turnpike
Syosset, NY 11791
(516) 364-5533
Provides free *Hands-On Health Care* catalog and information.

American Association of Acupuncture and Oriental Medicine
433 Front St.
Catasauqua, PA 18032
(610) 433-2448
Please send SASE for information on practitioners.

American Academy of Medical Acupuncturists
5820 Wilshire Blvd., Suite 500
Los Angeles, CA 90036
(213) 937-5514

ALEXANDER TECHNIQUE

American Center for the Alexander Technique
129 W. 67th St.
New York, NY 10002
(212) 799-0468

North American Society of the Teachers of Alexander Technique
P.O. Box 3992
Champaign, IL 61826
(800) 473-0620

AROMATHERAPY

The American Society for Phytotherapy and Aromatherapy International
P.O. Box 3679
South Pasadena, CA 91031
(818) 457-1742
Nonprofit organization; networking service; provides information.

International Society of Professional Aromatherapists
% Hinkley and District Hospital and Health Center
The Annex, Mount Road
Hinkley, Leics LE10 1AG England

BIOFEEDBACK

Biofeedback Certification Institute of America
10200 W. 44th Ave., Suite 304
Wheatridge, CO 80033
(303) 420-2902
Please send SASE for information and names of practitioners.

Life Sciences Institute of Mind/Body Health
2955 SW Wanamaker Drive, Suite B
Topeka, KS 66614
Provides outpatient program and general information.

HOW TO CHOOSE A BIOFEEDBACK THERAPIST

- Look for an individual who is licensed to practice independently or under the supervision of a licensed professional. Most biofeedback therapists are also psychologists; some are physicians, nurses, physical therapists, or other health-care professionals.
- An individual who has a certificate issued by the Biofeedback Certification Institute of America has passed the institute's high standards for training, experience, and education. Therapists without the certificate certainly may be as qualified as those with it.
- Choose a therapist who has worked with your type of headache. If the therapist hasn't worked with thermal biofeedback, for example, and you have migraine, you may want to find a therapist who has experience.
- Does the therapist answer all your questions? Do you feel comfortable asking them, or are you made to feel ignorant? Your comfort is critical; the last thing you need is more stress. If you do not feel at ease, find another therapist.

CHI KUNG

The Chi-Kung School
2730 29th St.
Boulder, CO 80301
(303) 442-3131

CHIROPRACTIC

The American Chiropractic Association
1701 Clarendon Blvd.
Arlington, VA 22209
(703) 276-8800

International Chiropractors Association
1110 N. Glebe Rd., Suite 1000
Arlington, VA 22201
(703) 528-5000

HOW TO CHOOSE A CHIROPRACTOR

According to the American Chiropractic Association, evaluate a chiropractor
(D.C., doctor of chiropractic) for the following. Does he or she:

- seem to be concerned about you as an individual?
- have a clean, neat office?
- provide emergency care?
- provide another chiropractor to take calls if he/she is away?
- explain the necessity for all exams and therapy and justify the need for
  treatment?
- tell you about the treatment before doing it and get your permission to
  do it?
- explain how many visits may be necessary? (If treatment is going to help,
  you should feel bettter within 4–6 weeks.)

Remember: Most chiropractors are not medical doctors; therefore, they are
not licensed to perform surgery or prescribe medications. Some, however, are
both M.D.'s and D.C.'s.

CRANIOSACRAL THERAPY

Colorado Cranial Institute
466 Marine St.
Boulder, CO 80302
(303) 447-2760

American Academy of Osteopathy
P.O. Box 750
Newark, OH 43055
(614) 349-8701

The Cranial Academy
3500 Depaw Blvd.
Indianapolis, IN 46268
(317) 879-0713
Please send SASE for information.

DIET/NUTRITION

American College of Nutrition
722 Robert E. Lee Dr.
Wilmington, NC 28412
(919) 452-1222
Provides help in finding a licensed nutritionist.

The Nutrition Action Health Letter Center for Science in the Public Interest
1875 Connecticut Ave. NW, Suite 300
Washington, DC 20009-5728
(202) 332-9111
Educates the general public about all areas of diet.

Vegetarian Resource Group
P.O. Box 1463
Baltimore, MD 21203
(410) 366-8343
Goal: to educate the public on health, nutrition, and the environment;
    publishes *The Vegetarian Journal.*

ENVIRONMENTAL MEDICINE

American Academy of Environmental Medicine (AAEM)
P.O. Box 16106
Denver, CO 80216
(303) 622-9755
Provides information about physicians in your area who specialize in
    environmental illness.

Nontoxic Hotline
(408) 684-0199
Provides information on allergy products and environmental resources.

Immuno Laboratories, Inc.
1620 West Oakland Park Blvd.
Fort Lauderdale, FL 33311
(800) 231-9197
Specializes in allergy (ELISA) and immunological testing.

Meridian Valley Clinical Laboratory (ELISA)
(800) 234-6825

Serammune Physicians Lab (ELISA ACT)
(800) 553-5472

FELDENKRAIS METHOD

Feldenkrais Guild
P.O. Box 489
Albany, OR 97321
(503) 926-0981

The Feldenkrais Foundation
P.O. Box 70157
Washington, DC 20088
(301) 656-1548

HERBAL MEDICINE

American Botanical Council
P.O. Box 201660
Austin, TX 78720
(800) 373-7105

Herb Society of America
9019 Kirtland Chardon Rd.
Kirtland, OH 44094
(216) 256-0514

HOMEOPATHY

Homeopathic Educational Services
2124 Kittredge St.
Berkeley, CA 94704
(510) 649-0294

International Foundation for Homeopathy
2366 Eastlake Ave., E 301
Seattle, WA 98102
(206) 776-4147
Provides general information on how to find practitioners in your area.

Homeopathic Academy of Naturopathic Physicians
14653 Graves Rd.
Mulino, OR 97042
(503) 795-0579

HYPNOSIS

Society for Clinical and Experimental Hypnosis
2200 E. Devon Ave., Suite 291
Des Plaines, IL 60018
(708) 297-3317
Please send SASE for information.

MACROBIOTICS

George Ohsawa Macrobiotic Foundation
1511 Robinson St.
Oroville, CA 95965

MEDITATION/VISUALIZATION

Mind-Body Medical Institute
New Deaconess Hospital, Harvard Medical School
Boston, MA 02215
(617) 632-9530

Psycho-Acoustic Technology
4536 Genoa Circle
Virginia Beach, VA 23462
(804) 456-9487

The Institute of Transpersonal Psychology
744 San Antonio Rd.
Palo Alto, CA 94303
(415) 493-4430
Imagery training; certification program in mind–body consciousness.

The Academy for Guided Imagery
P.O. Box 2070
Mill Valley, CA 94942
(800) 726-2070

MYOTHERAPY

Bonnie Prudden Pain Erasure
3661 N. Campbell, Suite 102
Tucson, AZ 85719
(800) 221-4643

ORIENTAL MASSAGE

The Amma Institute
1596 Post St.
San Francisco, CA 94109

OSTEOPATHY

Look under "D.O., Doctor of Osteopathy," in the "Physicians" section of the
Yellow Pages.

American Osteopathic Association
142 E. Ontario St.
Chicago, IL 60611
(312) 280-5800
Provides information and names of practitioners in your area.

American Osteopathic Academy of Sclerotherapy
107 Maple Ave.
Wilmington, DE 19809
(302) 792-9280

PHYSICAL THERAPY

Look for a licensed professional. At least 30 states allow people to be treated by a physical therapist without a referral from a physician. Contact local hospitals, colleges with physical therapy programs, your state association of physical therapists, or:

The American Physical Therapy Association
1111 N. Fairfax St.
Alexandria, VA 22314
(703) 684-2782

POLARITY THERAPY

American Polarity Therapy Association
2888 Bluff St., Suite 149
Boulder, CO 80301
(303) 545-2080

REFLEXOLOGY

International Institute of Reflexology
P.O. Box 12642
St. Petersburg, FL 33733-2642
(813) 343-4811
Provides information, seminars, training, books, and referrals.

SWEDISH MASSAGE

American Massage Therapy Association
1130 West North Shore Ave.
Chicago, IL 60626
(312) 761-AMTA

YOGA

International Association of Yoga Therapists
109 Hillside Ave.
Mill Valley, CA 94941
(415) 383-4587
Nonprofit organization that focuses on research on and education about yoga.

PAIN CENTERS OR CLINICS AND STRESS CENTERS

The goals of pain centers (inpatient) or clinics (outpatient) are to help individuals (1) take more responsibility for their health, (2) become more functional, (3) improve their comfort level, (4) decrease or eliminate their dependence on medication, and (5) have more control of their pain. Stress centers help individuals learn stress reduction techniques and incorporate them into their lives.

TYPES OF PAIN FACILITIES

1. *Unidiscipline:* The physician or other health-care professional(s) practices one specialty, such as neurology.
2. *Interdiscipline:* At least one physician on staff who interacts with other health-care professionals (occupational therapists, physical therapists, and so on) as part of a treatment team.
3. *Multidiscipline:* Two or more physicians from different specialties who work with other health-care professionals.
4. *Comprehensive pain center:* Offers both inpatient and outpatient care.
5. *Syndrome-oriented program:* A facility that treats one kind of pain, such as headache, back pain, cancer, and so on.
6. *Modality-oriented program:* A facility that offers one kind of therapy, for example: acupuncture, physical therapy, or transcutaneous electrical nerve stimulation (TENS).

The following is a representative list of the many mind-body clinics and/ or stress-reduction clinics in the United States.

The American Institute of Stress
124 Park Ave.
Yonkers, NY 10703
(800) 24-RELAX
Provides information about mind-body relationships; publishes newsletter.

Stress Reduction Clinic
Jon Kabat-Zinn, Ph.D.
P.O. Box 547
University of Massachusetts Medical Center
Lexington, MA 02173
(508) 856-2656
Largest hospital-based stress reduction clinic in the United States.

Stress Reduction Clinic
University of Massachusetts Medical Center
Worcester, MA 01655
(508) 856-1616

Life Transition Therapy
110 Delgado Compound, Suite A
Santa Fe, NM 87501
(505) 982-4183

Mind/Body Medicine Clinic
2440 East Fifth St.
Tyler, TX 75701
(903) 592-2202

Stress Reduction Clinic
Rehabilitation Institute of Pittsburgh
6301 Northumberland St.
Pittsburgh, PA 15217
(412) 521-9000

APPENDIX II

Contacts for Natural Therapy Supplies

Here are some resources for cassettes, videos, and magazines about natural therapies as well as sources for herbs, homeopathic remedies, and other natural therapy items. Contact these companies for their catalog or for more information on their products.

AROMATHERAPY

Aromaland
Rte. 20, Box 29AL
Santa Fe, NM 87501

Aroma Vera
5901 Rodeo Rd.
Los Angeles, CA 90016
(310) 280-0407

Essence Aromatherapy
P.O. Box 2119
Durango, CO 81302
(800) 283-0244

Santa Fe Fragrance
P.O. Box 282
Santa Fe, NM 87504
(505) 473-1717

Aromatic Concepts
12629 N. Tatum Blvd., Suite 611
Phoenix, AZ 85032
(602) 861-3696

Original Swiss Aromatics
P.O. Box 6842
San Rafael, CA 95904
(415) 459-3998

The Body Shop
45 Horsehill Rd.
Cedar Knolls, NJ 07927
(800) 451-2535

DIET AND NUTRITION

The Nutrition Action Health Letter
Center for Science in the Public Interest
1875 Connecticut Ave. NW, Suite 300
Washington, DC 20009-5728
(202) 332-9111
Publishes a monthly newsletter for the general public; covers dietary
   information, reviews books and recipes.

Vegetarian Journal
Vegetarian Resource Group
P.O. Box 1463
Baltimore, MD 21203
(410) 366-8343
Nonprofit group, whose mission is to educate the public about health,
   nutrition, and the environment; publishes a journal.

Vegetarian Voice
North American Vegetarian Society
P.O. Box 72
Dolgeville, NY 13329
Nonprofit group publishes a bimonthly journal. Focus is on health,
   compassionate living, and the environment; contains recipes.

Vegetarian Times
P.O. Box 570
Oak Park, IL 60303
(708) 848-8100
Monthly publication with many articles on health, nutrition, and cooking.

ENVIRONMENTAL MEDICINE

Dr. Rogers & Environmental Illness Recovery (videotape)
Robin Kormos Productions
149 Avenue A
New York, NY 10009-8921

FELDENKRAIS METHOD

Feldenkrais Resources
(800) 765-1907
Home programs on audiotape by authorized publisher of Dr. Feldenkrais's
   work.

Relaxercise
(800) 735-7950
Audiotapes based on Dr. Feldenkrais's work.

HERBS

East Earth Herb Inc.
P.O. Box 802
Eugene, OR 97402
(800) 827-HERB

The Herb Closet
104 Main St.
Montpelier, VT 05602
(802) 223-0888

Jean's Greens
R.R. 1, Box 55J
Rensselaerville, NY 12147
(518) 239-8327

Mountain Rose Herbs
P.O. Box 2000
Redway, CA 95560
(707) 923-7867

Nature's Way
10 Mountain Springs Parkway
Springville, UT 84663
Products available in stores.

OSO Herbals
P.O. Box 50306-278
Tucson, AZ 85703
(520) 624-9225

Terra Firma Botanicals
28653 Sutherlin Lane
Eugene, OR 97405
Fresh and dried herbal extracts; massage oils; catalog.

HOMEOPATHY

Boericke & Tafel, Inc.
Santa Rose, CA 95407
(800) 876-9505
The oldest homeopathic pharmaceutical firm in the United States.

Homeopathic Overnight
4111 Simon Rd.
Youngstown, OH 44512
(800) ARNICA30
Mail-order homeopathic remedies.

Homeopathic Educational Services
2124 Kittredge St.
Berkeley, CA 94704
(510) 649-0294 information; (800) 359-9051 orders only
Catalog of remedies, books, tapes, and cassettes.

Hadas Natural Products Ltd.
P.O. Box 48059
Atlanta, GA 30362
(800) 99-HADAS for information and mail orders.
Extensive line of homeopathic remedies. Also look for them in your pharmacy.

HORMONE TESTING

Aeron Life Cycles
(800) 631-7900

Diagnos-Techs Inc.
(800) 878-3787

MASSAGE

Royal Pyramid, Inc.
414 Manhattan Ave.
Hawthorne, NY 10532
(800) 325-7423
Ask for their catalog of massage supplies and accessories.

Massage Magazine
P.O. Box 1500
Davis, CA 95617
(916) 757-6033
Bimonthly; covers massage, bodywork, and related healing arts.

MEDITATION/VISUALIZATION TAPES

QuantumQuests
Box 986
Oakview, CA 93022
(800) 772-0090

High-Tech Meditation
(800) 962-2033

Health Journeys, available on Time Warner AudioBooks: *For People with
    Headaches* (two-tape set).
Tapes by Belleruth Naparstek, Image Paths, Inc.
2635 Payne Ave.
Cleveland, OH 44114
(800) 800-8661

The Source Cassette Learning System
Emmet Miller, M.D.
945 Evelyn St.
Menlo Park, CA 94025
(415) 328-7171
Offers tapes for relaxation, pain relief; free catalog.

MindBody Health Sciences
22 Lawson Terrace
Scituate, MA 02066
(617) 545-7122
Offers books and tapes for mental health applications.

MOVEMENT THERAPY

The MEND Clinic
9121 Tanque Verde #105
Tucson, AZ 85749
(520) 749-0800
Videocassettes and audiocassettes available.

SYNAPTIC MACHINE

U.S. Medical Sales, Inc.
6549 S. Xerophon Street
Littleton, CO 80127
(800) 607-7455

YOGA

Himalayan Institute of Yoga, Science, and Philosophy
R.R. 1 Box 400
Honesdale, PA 18431
(717) 253-5551
Catalog of books, videos, and tapes; holds classes and has centers around the
    country. Also publishes the magazine *Yoga International*.

Samata Yoga and Health Institute
4150 Tivoli Ave.
Los Angeles, CA 90066
(310) 306-8845
Manuals, videos, and audiocassettes available; classes also.

Total Yoga (video)
White Lotus Foundation
(805) 964-1944
Call for information.

Yoga for Beginners (video)
Patricia Walden, Rudra Press
(800) 394-6286
Call for their 75-minute video for beginning hatha yoga.

Tools for Yoga
(201) 966-5311
Call for their catalog.

Yoga Props
(415) 285-9642
Call for their catalog.

SOURCES AND SUGGESTED READINGS

GENERAL

Benson, Herbert. *The Wellness Book.* New York: Carol Publishing Group, 1992.

Berkow, Robert, M.D., ed. *Merck Manual*, vol. I. Rahway, NJ: Merck, Sharp and Dohme, 1992.

Bland, Jeffrey S., Ph.D. *Applying New Essentials in Nutritional Medicine.* Gig Harbor, WA: Health Communications, 1995.

Carroll, David. *The Complete Book of Natural Medicine.* New York: Simon & Schuster, 1980.

Diamond, Seymour, and Donald Dalessio. *The Practicing Physician's Approach to Headache,* 5th ed. Baltimore: Williams & Wilkins, 1992.

Ehrmantrant, Harry C., Ph.D. *Headaches: The Drugless Way to Lasting Relief.* Berkeley, CA: Celestial Arts, 1987.

Feiss, George. *Mind Therapies, Body Therapies.* Millbrae, CA: Celestial Arts, 1979.

Goddard, Greg, D.D.S. *TMJ—The Jaw Connection, The Overlooked Diagnosis.* Santa Fe, NM: Aurora Press, 1991.

Golan, Ralph, M.D. *Optimal Wellness.* New York: Ballantine, 1995.

Hafen, Brent, and Kathryn Frandsen. *From Acupuncture to Yoga.* Englewood Cliffs, NJ: Prentice Hall, 1983.

Inglis, Brian, and Ruth West. *Alternative Health Guide.* New York: Knopf, 1992.

Isselbacher, Kurt J. et al. *Harrison's Principles of Internal Medicine,* 13th ed. New York: McGraw-Hill, 1995.

Kahn, Ada P. *Headaches.* New York: Contemporary Books, 1983.

Kastner, Mark. *Alternative Healing: The Complete A–Z Guide to Over 160 Different Alternative Therapies.* La Mesa, CA: Halcyon Publishers, 1993.

Lance, James W. *Mechanism and Management of Headache,* 5th ed. London: Butterworth-Heinemann, 1993.

Pizzorno, Joseph E., and Michael T. Murray. *A Textbook of Natural Medicine.* Seattle: John Bastyr College Publications, 1988.

Prevention editors. *Hands-On Healing.* Emmaus, PA: Rodale Press, 1989.

Rakel, Robert E., M.D., ed. *Conn's Current Therapy.* Philadelphia: WB Saunders, 1994.

Rapoport, Alan M., and Fred D. Sheftell. *Headache Relief.* New York: Simon & Schuster, 1990.

Raskin, Neil Hugh. *Headache,* 2d ed. New York: Churchill Livingstone, 1988.

Robbins, Lawrence, M.D., and Susan S. Lang. *Headache Help.* Boston: Houghton Mifflin, 1995.

Smyth, Angela. *The Complete Home Healer.* New York: HarperCollins, 1994.

Solomon, Seymour, and Fraccaro. *The Headache Book.* Yonkers, NY: Consumer Reports Book, 1991.

Stoff, Jesse A., M.D., and Charles R. Pellegrino, Ph.D. *Chronic Fatigue Syndrome: The Hidden Epidemic.* New York: Harper Perennial, 1990.

Thomas, Clayton L., M.D., ed. *Taber's Cyclopedic Medical Dictionary,* 16th ed. Philadelphia: FA Davis, 1989.

Trattler, Ross. *Better Health Through Natural Healing.* New York: McGraw-Hill, 1988.

Weil, Andrew. *Natural Health, Natural Medicine.* Boston: Houghton-Mifflin, 1990.

Whitaker, Julian, M.D. *Dr. Whitaker's Guide to Natural Healing.* Rocklin, CA: Prima Publishing, 1995.

Wilson, Jean D. et al. *Principles of Internal Medicine,* 12th ed. New York: McGraw-Hill, 1991.

ACUPRESSURE

Bauer, Cathryn. *Acupressure for Everyone.* New York: Henry Holt, 1991.

Gach, Michael Reed. *Acupressure's Potent Points: A Guide to Self-Care for Common Ailments.* New York: Bantam, 1994.

Houston, F. M. *The Healing Benefits of Acupressure,* rev. ed. New Canaan, CT: Keats, 1994.

Kenyon, Keith, M.D. *Pressure Points: Do-It-Yourself Acupuncture Without Needles.* New York: Arco Publishing, 1984.

Lundberg, Paul. *The Book of Shiatsu.* London: Gaia Books, 1992.

Nickel, David J. *Acupressure for Athletes.* New York: Henry Holt, 1987.

Ohashi, Wataru. *Do-It-Yourself Shiatsu.* New York: Viking, 1992.

Serizawa, Katsusuke, M.D. *Tsubo: Vital Points for Oriental Therapy.* New York: Japan Publications, 1976.

ACUPUNCTURE

Chaitow, Leon. *The Acupuncture Treatment of Pain: Safe and Effective Methods.* Rochester, VT: Healing Arts, 1990.

Marcus, Paul. *Acupuncture: A Patient's Guide.* New York: Thorsons, 1985.

Marcus, Paul. *Thorsons Introductory Guide to Acupuncture.* London: Hammersmith, 1991.

Stux, Gabriel. *Basics of Acupuncture.* Berlin, New York: Springer-Verlag, 1988.

AROMATHERAPY

Berwick, Ann. *Holistic Aromatherapy*. St. Paul, MN: Llewellyn Publications, 1994.

Cunningham, S. *Magical Aromatherapy*. St. Paul, MN: Llewellyn Publications, 1989.

Jackson, Judith. *Scentual Touch: A Personal Guide to Aromatherapy*. New York: Ballantine Books, 1986.

Price, Shirley. *Aromatherapy for Common Ailments*. New York: Simon & Schuster, 1991.

Rechelbacher, Horst. *Rejuvenation: A Wellness Guide for Women and Men*. Rochester, VT: Inner Traditions International, 1987.

Tisserand, Robert. *Aromatherapy: To Heal and Tend the Body*. Wilmot, WI: Lotus Press, 1988.

Tisserand, Robert. *The Art of Aromatherapy: The Healing and Beautifying Properties of the Essential Oils of Flowers and Herbs*. Rochester, VT: Inner Traditions International, 1987.

Wildwood, Christine. *Holistic Aromatherapy*. Wellingborough, UK: Thorsons, 1986.

Worwood, Valerie. *The Complete Book of Essential Oils and Aromatherapy*. New York: New World Library, 1991.

BIOFEEDBACK

Green, Elmer. *Beyond Biofeedback*. New York: Delacorte, 1977.

Sedlacek, Kurt. *The Sedlacek Technique: Finding the Calm*. New York: McGraw-Hill, 1989.

CHI KUNG

Chang, Simon, and Fritz Pokorny. *Easy Tao*. San Francisco: China Books, 1988.

China Sports magazine. *The Wonders of Qigong*. Los Angeles: Wayfarer Publishers, 1985.

Jwing-Ming, Yang. *The Essence of Tai Chi Chi Kung*. Jamaica Plain, MA: Yang Martial Arts Association, 1990.

Jwing-Ming, Yang. *The Root of Chinese Chi Yung*. Jamaica Plain, MA: Yang Martial Arts Association, 1987.

CHIROPRACTIC

Altman, Nathaniel. *Everybody's Guide to Chiropractic Health Care*. Los Angeles: Jeremy P. Tarcher, 1990.

Holmquist, Karl. *Home Chiropractic Handbook*. Forks, WA: One 8 Inc., 1985.

DIET AND NUTRITION

Balch, James F., and Phyllis A. Balch. *Prescription for Nutritional Healing*. Garden City Park, NY: Avery Publishing, 1990.

Ballentine, Rudolph. *Transition to Vegetarianism: An Evolutionary Step.* Honesdale, PA: Himalayan Publishers, 1987.

Colbin, Annemarie. *Food and Healing.* New York: Ballantine, 1986.

Gagne, Steve. *The Energetics of Food.* Santa Fe, NM: Spiral Sciences, 1990.

Haas, Elson M., M.D. *Staying Healthy with Nutrition.* Berkeley, CA: Celestial Arts, 1992.

Klaper, Michael, M.D. *Vegan Nutrition Pure and Simple.* Maui, HI: Gentle World, 1987.

Lappe, Frances M. *Diet for a Small Planet,* rev. ed. New York: Ballantine Books, 1975.

Ohsawa, George. *The Art of Peace.* Oroville, CA: George Ohsawa Macrobiotic Foundation, 1990.

Pickarski, Ron. *Friendly Foods.* Berkeley, CA: Ten Speed Press, 1991.

Robbins, John. *Diet for a New America: How Your Food Choices Affect Your Health, Happiness, and the Future of Life on Earth.* Walpole, NH: Stillpoint Publishing, 1987.

Robbins, John. *May All Be Fed.* New York: Morrow, 1992; Avon, 1993.

Wasserman, Debbie. *Simply Vegan: Quick Vegetarian Meals.* Baltimore: Vegetarian Resource Group, 1991.

Werbach, Melvyn, M.D. *Healing with Food.* New York: Harper Perennial, 1993.

DRUGS/MEDICATIONS

Griffith, H. Winter, M.D. *Complete Guide to Prescription and Nonprescription Drugs,* 1995 ed. New York: Berkley Publishing Group, 1994.

Monthly Prescribing Reference. New York: Prescribing Reference, January 1995.

1996 Physicians GenRx. St. Louis: Mosby Year Book, 1996.

Schein, Jeffrey, and Philip Hansten. *Consumer's Guide to Drug Interactions.* New York: Collier Books, 1993.

United States Pharmacopeial Convention, Inc. *About Your Medicines.* Rockville, MD: United States Pharmacopeial Convention, 1993.

Winter, Ruth. *A Consumer's Dictionary of Medicines.* New York: Crown Publishers, 1993.

ENVIRONMENTAL MEDICINE

Breecher, Maury M., and Shirley Linde. *Healthy Homes in a Toxic World.* New York: John Wiley, 1992.

Randolph, Theron C., M.D., and Ralph W. Moss, Ph.D. *An Alternative Approach to Allergies.* New York: HarperCollins, 1990.

Rogers, Sherry A., M.D. *The E.I. Syndrome: Environmental Illness.* Syracuse, NY: Prestige, 1995.

Rogers, Sherry A., M.D. *Tired or Toxic.* Syracuse, NY: Prestige, 1990.

Rogers, Sherry A., M.D. *Chemical Sensitivity.* Edited by Don R. Benson. New Canaan, CT: Keats, 1995.

HERBAL MEDICINE

Carroll, David. *The Complete Book of Natural Medicine*. New York: Summit Books, 1980.

Castleman, Michael. *The Healing Herbs*. Emmaus, PA: Rodale Press, 1991.

Elias, Jason, and Shelagh Masline. *Healing Herbal Remedies*. New York: Dell, 1995.

Hoffman, David. *An Herbal Guide to Stress Relief*. Rochester, VT: Healing Arts Press, 1991.

Inglis, Brian, and Ruth West. *The Alternative Health Guide*. New York: Knopf, 1983.

Lucas, Richard M. *Miracle Medicine Herbs*. Englewood Cliffs, NJ: Prentice-Hall, 1990.

Mills, Simon, and Steven Finando. *Alternatives in Healing*. New York: NAL Books, 1989.

Mindell, Earl, R.Ph., Ph.D. *Earl Mindell's Herb Bible*. New York: Simon & Schuster, 1992.

Moore, Michael. *Medicinal Plants of the Desert and Canyon West*. Santa Fe, NM: Museum of New Mexico Press, 1989.

Murray, Michael T., N.D. *The Healing Power of Herbs*. Rocklin, CA: Prima Publishing, 1991.

Murray, Michael T., N.D. *Natural Alternatives to Over-the-Counter and Prescription Drugs*. New York: William Morrow, 1994.

Sherman, John A., N.D. *The Complete Botanical Prescriber*. Compiled by John A. Sherman, N.D., 1993.

Stein, Diane. *All Women Are Healers*. Freedom, CA: The Crossing Press, 1990.

Tierra, Lesley. *The Herbs of Life: Health and Healing Using Western and Chinese Techniques*. Freedom, CA: The Crossing Press, 1992.

Tierra, Michael, N.D. *Planetary Herbology*. Twin Lakes, WI: Lotus Press, 1988.

Tierra, Michael, N.D. *The Way of Herbs*. New York: Simon & Schuster, 1990.

Trattler, Ross. *Better Health Through Natural Healing*. New York: McGraw-Hill, 1985.

HOMEOPATHY

Blackie, Margery G. *The Patient Not the Cure: The Challenge of Homeopathy*. Macdonald & Jane's, 1976.

Coulter, C. *Portraits of Homeopathic Medicine*. 2 vols. Berkeley: North Atlantic Books, 1986.

Cummings, Stephen, and Dana Ullman. *Everybody's Guide to Homeopathic Medicine*. Los Angeles: Jeremy P. Tarcher, 1991.

Gibson, D. M. *Studies of Homeopathic Remedies*. Beaconsfield, England: Beaconsfield Publishers, 1987.

Hahnemann, Samuel. *The Organon of Medicine*. Translated by J. Kunli, A. Naude, and P. Pendleton. London: Gollancz, 1986.

Koehler, Gerhard. *The Handbook of Homeopathy*. San Francisco: Thorsons Publishing Group, 1986.

Lockie, Andrew. *The Home Guide to Homeopathy*. New York: Simon & Schuster, 1989, 1993.

Mills, Simon, and Steven J. Finando. *Alternatives in Healing*. New York: New American Library, 1988.

Panos, Maesimund B. *Homeopathic Medicine at Home*. Los Angeles: Jeremy P. Tarcher, 1980.

Rose, Barry. *The Family Health Guide to Homeopathy*. Berkeley, CA: Celestial Arts, 1992.

Stephenson, James H. *A Doctor's Guide to Helping Yourself with Homeopathic Remedies*, 1st British ed. Wellingborough, England: Thorsons Publishers, 1977.

Ullman, Dana. *Homeopathy: Medicine for the 21st Century*. Berkeley, CA: North Atlantic Books, 1988.

Weiner, Michael. *The Complete Book of Homeopathy*. Garden City, NY: Avery Publishing Group, 1989.

Weinstein, Corey, and Nancy Bruning. *Healing Homeopathic Remedies*. New York: Dell, 1996.

HYPNOSIS

Copelan, Rachael. *How to Hypnotize Yourself and Others*. New York: Bell Publishing, 1984.

Fisher, Stanley. *Discovering the Power of Self-Hypnosis*. New York: Harper-Collins, 1991.

Haley, Jay. *Uncommon Therapy*. New York: WW Norton, 1987.

Hilgad, Ernest. *Hypnosis: In the Relief of Pain*. New York: Brunner/Mazel, 1994.

Miller, Michael M.D. *Therapeutic Hypnosis*. New York: Human Sciences Press, 1979.

Wallace, Benjamin. *Applied Hypnosis*. Chicago: Nelson-Hall, 1979.

Yates, John. *The Complete Book of Self-Hypnosis*. Chicago: Nelson-Hall, 1984.

MASSAGE

Anhui Medical School, China. *Chinese Massage*. Point Roberts, WA: Hartley & Marks, 1987.

Inkeles, Gordon. *The Art of Sensual Massage*. New York: Simon & Schuster, 1974.

Kaptchuk, Ted. *The Web That Has No Weaver: Understanding Chinese Medicine*. Congdon & Weed, 1993.

Lidell, Lucinda et al. *The Book of Massage*. New York: Simon & Schuster, 1984.

Ravald, Bertild. *The Art of Swedish Massage*. New York: EP Dutton, 1984.

Tappan, Frances M. *Healing Massage Techniques*. Appleton & Lange, 1988.

MEDITATION/VISUALIZATION/RELAXATION

Achterberg, Jeanne. *Rituals of Healing: Using Imagery for Health and Wellness*. New York: Bantam, 1994.

Benson, Herbert, M.D. *The Relaxation Response*. New York: Morrow & Co., 1975.

Benson, Herbert, M.D. *Your Maximum Mind*. New York: Time Books, 1987.

Borysenko, Joan. *Minding the Body, Mending the Mind*. New York: Bantam, 1987.

Dachman, Ken, and John Lyons. *You Can Relieve Pain: How Guided Imagery Can Help You Reduce Pain or Eliminate It Altogether.* New York: Harper & Row, 1990.

Dass, Ram. *Journey of Awakening: A Meditator's Guidebook.* New York: Bantam, 1978.

Epstein, Gerald, M.D. *Healing Visualizations.* New York: Bantam, 1989.

Fanning, Patrick. *Visualization for Change.* Oakland, CA: New Harbinger, 1988.

Goldstein, Joseph, and Jack Kornfield. *Seeking the Heart of Wisdom.* Boston: Shambhala, 1987.

Kabat-Zinn, Jon. *Wherever You Go, There You Are: Mindfulness Meditation in Everyday Life.* New York: Hyperion, 1994.

Levey, Joel. *The Fine Arts of Relaxation, Concentration, and Meditation.* London: Wisdom Publications, 1987.

McDonald, Kathleen. *How to Meditate: A Practical Guide.* London: Wisdom Publications, 1992.

Naparstek, Belleruth. *Staying Well with Guided Imagery.* New York: Time Warner, 1994.

Rossman, Martin. *Healing Yourself: A Step-by-Step Program for Better Health Through Imagery.* New York: Walker, 1987.

Speads, Carola. *Ways to Better Breathing.* Rochester, VT: Inner Traditions, 1992.

Suzuki, Shunryu. *Zen Mind, Beginner's Mind.* New York: Weatherhill, 1987.

MIND/BODY

Chopra, Deepak, M.D. *Perfect Health: The Complete Mind/Body Guide.* New York: Harmony Books, 1991.

Chopra, Deepak, M.D. *Quantum Healing: Exploring the Frontiers of the Body, Mind, Medicine.* Bantam, 1993.

Cousins, Norman. *Anatomy of an Illness as Perceived by the Patient.* New York: Norton, 1979.

Cousins, Norman. *Head First: The Biology of Hope and the Healing Power of the Human Spirit.* New York: Viking, 1990.

Dienstfrey, Harris. *Where the Mind Meets the Body.* New York: HarperCollins, 1991.

Goleman, Daniel, and Joel Gurin. *Mind/Body Medicine.* Yonkers, NY: Consumer Reports Books, 1993.

Ornstein, Robert, and David Sobel. *The Healing Brain.* New York: Simon & Schuster, 1988.

Ornstein, Robert, and David Sobel. *Healthy Pleasures.* Reading, MA: Addison-Wesley, 1990.

Pelletier, Kenneth R. *Mind as Healer, Mind as Slayer,* rev. ed. New York: Delacorte, 1992.

Siegel, Bernie, M.D. *Love, Medicine and Miracles: Lessons Learned About Self-Healing From a Surgeon's Experience with Exceptional Patients.* Boston: GK Hall, 1988.

Siegel, Bernie, M.D. *Peace, Love and Healing: Bodymind Communication and the Path to Self-Healing.* New York: Harper & Row, 1989.

Weiss, Brian M.D. *Through Time into Healing*. New York: Simon & Schuster, 1992.

MYOTHERAPY

Prudden, Bonnie. *Myotherapy: Bonnie Prudden's Complete Guide to Pain-Free Living*. New York: Ballantine, 1980.
Prudden, Bonnie. *Pain-Erasure: The Bonnie Prudden Way*. New York: Ballantine, 1980.

POSTURE

Alexander, F. M. *Constructive Conscious Control of the Individual*. Long Beach, CA: Centerline Press, 1985.
Alexander, F. M. *Use of the Self*. London: Victor Gollanez, 1985.
Brennan, R. *The Alexander Workbook*. Shaftbury, England: Element Books, 1992.
Caplan, Deborah. *Back Trouble: A New Approach to Prevention and Recovery Based on the Alexander Technique*. Gainesville, FL: Triad Publishing, 1987.
Feldenkrais, Moshe. *Awareness Through Movement: Easy to Do Exercises to Improve Posture, Vision, Imagination and Personal Awareness*. San Francisco: Harper, 1991.
Feldenkrais, Moshe. *The Potent Self: A Guide to Spontaneity*. San Francisco: Harper, 1992.
Leibowitz, Judith, and Bill Connington. *The Alexander Technique*. New York: Harper & Row, 1990.
Pierce Jones, Frank. *Body Awareness in Action*. New York: Schocken Books, 1976.
Steven G. *Alexander Technique*. London: Macdonald Optima, 1991.

POLARITY THERAPY

Beaulieu, John. *Polarity Therapy Workbook*. 1994. Contact the Polarity Wellness Center, 10 Leonard Street, New York, NY 10013.
Stone, Randolph. *Health Building*. Sebastopol, CA: CRCS Publishing, 1985.
Teschler, Wilfried. *The Polarity Healing Handbook*. Bath, England: Gateway Books and San Leandro, CA: Interbook, 1986.

REFLEXOLOGY

Byers, Dwight. *Better Health with Foot Reflexology*. Available through the International Institute of Reflexology, P.O. Box 12642, St. Petersburg, FL 33733-2642.
Kunz, Kevin, and Barbara Kunz. *Complete Guide to Foot Reflexology*, rev. ed. Englewood Cliffs, NJ: Prentice-Hall, 1991.
Kunz, Kevin, and Barbara Kunz. *Hand and Foot Reflexology: A Self-Help Guide*. Englewood Cliffs, NJ: Prentice-Hall, 1984.
Norman, Laura. *Feet First: A Guide to Foot Reflexology*. New York: Simon & Schuster, 1988.

THERAPEUTIC TOUCH

Cohen, Sherry. *The Magic of Touch*. New York: Harper & Row, 1987.

Krieger, Dolores. *The Therapeutic Touch: How to Use Your Hands to Help and to Heal*. Englewood Cliffs, NJ: Prentice-Hall, 1979.

Macrae, Janet. *Therapeutic Touch: A Practical Guide*. New York: Knopf, 1988.

YOGA

Folan, Lilias. *Yoga and Your Life*. New York: Macmillan, 1981.

Hewitt, James. *The Complete Yoga Book*. New York: Schocken Books, 1978.

Kundalini Research Institute. *Sadhana Guidelines for Kundalina Yoga Daily Practice*. Los Angeles: Arcline Publications, 1988.

Sivananda Yoga Vedanta Center. *Learn Yoga in a Weekend*. New York: Knopf, 1993.

INDEX

In this index, page numbers in italic type indicate text in boxes and figures.

ABOUT THE AUTHORS

Paula Maas, D.O., M.D. (H.), is Clinical Medical Director and Clinical Administrator of the MEND CLINIC in Tucson, Arizona, a multidisciplinary team of practitioners who provide coordinated care in nutritional therapy, acupuncture, naturopathy (including herbal therapy), homeopathy, biofeedback, and stress reduction. At the same time, Dr. Maas also retains strong professional ties to the more mainstream medical community, maintaining hospital privileges at St. Mary's and the Tucson Medical Center. Both Dr. Maas and the extensive network of complementary and traditional medicine professionals at her disposal offer a unique and rich resource for this book.

Dr. Maas also maintains a private family practice in Tucson and is Project Manager for the United States Health Information Network, a collaborative effort among private and government organizations to design a universally accessible, national network for health care information.

Dr. Maas speaks frequently to community and corporate groups about health issues, especially effective alternative treatment regimens in general and for women's health issues.

Dr. Maas is unusually well regarded by both the allopathic and alternative medical community. She is willing to use her considerable energies and resources to help promote and publicize these books.

Deborah Mitchell is a health and medical journalist who has written extensively for both the professional and lay audience. She most recently completed collaborating on two books for the Dell Caregiver's Library series, *The National Stroke Association's Guide to Stroke Recovery* and *When Your Loved One Has Alzheimer's*. She is also the author of *Natural Medicine for Diabetes*. Since 1987, she has published hundreds of articles and abstracts as a writer for professional publications. Her monthly column, "Medical Challenges," appears in Internal Medicine World Report, which reaches more than 100,000 medical practitioners.

ABOUT THE PRODUCER

Lynn Sonberg Book Services specializes in producing health, medical and nutrition titles for a general audience, including books that take an alternative approach to health problems. Among the sixty titles Ms. Sonberg has produced for major publishers are thirty-two titles in the Dell Medical Library and the Dell Caregiver's Library. These include ten books on women's health issues, ranging from infertility and osteoporosis to PMS and menopause. Other books on women's health include *Healing the Female Heart: A Holistic Approach to Prevention and Recovery from Heart Disease* by Elizabeth Ross, M.D., and Judith Sachs (Pocket). She is also responsible for *Healing Herbal Remedies* by Jason Elias and Shelagh Masline and *Healing Homeopathic Remedies* by Nancy Bruning and Corey Weinstein, M.D., forthcoming from Dell Publishing.